It was a pleasure to take care of J ⸻ ;o to
work and prepare for the unexp⸻ ⸻ unexpected
cases. Brain surgery and steroid p⸍,⸍⸍osis. It is a terrifying experience!
As a nurse you go into the trenches with your patient, and you fight for
their healing and safety while providing emotional comfort.

It brings me comfort to know that Joe is fully recovered and living
the life he deserves with his friends and family.

Bonnie Manchur RN., Brigham and Women's Hospital

Your book is a gift to those facing what others feel are insurmountable
odds for recovery. The power of perseverance, family, faith and the
miraculous hands of Dr. Black was paramount to your amazing
outcome. Thank you for sharing your story.

Bailey, Nancy D. Olsen, RN., to Dr. Peter Black

"This book is very emotional. Having Nancy and I be a part of the
journey is a blessing to help such wonderful people like you. We love
caring and guiding the way through the fear, life-changing moments
and the management of the medications." Some important points you
mentioned for anyone having to go through an unfortunate incident:

Have an advocate,

Seek more than one opinion,

Never give up,

Choose your doctor and hospital carefully,

Seek the best in everything, radiation is sometimes needed for 'benign'
tumors,

Choose your rehabilitation site carefully,

GET SUPPORT from the medical team, family and friends and your
medical/surgical journey will be better than without these elements.

Donna DelloIacono NP., to Dr. Peter Black

I Wiggled My Toes ... Hallelujah!

An Unforeseen Journey of Recovery from Brain Surgery

Reader,

Best of Health

Joe

November 20, 2021

Joseph C. Salvo

WESTBOW
P R E S S®
A DIVISION OF THOMAS NELSON
& ZONDERVAN

The author will donate a portion of the proceeds from the sale of the book to the American Brain Tumor Association.

WestBow Press books may be ordered through booksellers or by contacting:

WestBow Press
A Division of Thomas Nelson & Zondervan
1663 Liberty Drive
Bloomington, IN 47403
www.westbowpress.com
844-714-3454

Cover design by Christine Dupre, www.vidagraphicdesign.com
Photo of Dr. Peter Black by Susan R. Symonds for Mainframe Photographics

Scripture taken from the King James Version of the Bible.

ISBN: 978-1-6642-2252-6 (sc)
ISBN: 978-1-6642-2253-3 (hc)
ISBN: 978-1-6642-2251-9 (e)

Library of Congress Control Number: 2021902128

Print information available on the last page.

WestBow Press rev. date: 04/22/2021

CONTENTS

DEDICATION -

This book is dedicated to eight individuals who are, and will always be, very special to me: my Mother, Angie; my Father, Harry; my sister, Patty; my brothers Skip and Chris; world-renowned surgeon Dr. Peter Black; wonderful friend Ann Ormond, former Director of Marketing and Community and Public Relations at Waltham Hospital; and family friend and spiritual confidant Father Charles Egan, pastor of our closely knit Sacred Heart parish.

FOREWORD

by Dr. Peter Black
Medical Note

Introduction

This is an extraordinary book by an extraordinary person. The account Joe Salvo gives us of his recuperation from meningioma surgery provides a rare opportunity to experience postoperative recovery from a patient's perspective. As Mr. Salvo says, the story demonstrates that "with determination and hard work, anything is possible."

It is a pleasure to add a few words to his introduction. Comments on meningiomas, surgery, steroid psychosis, family, faith, and determination seem relevant.

Meningiomas. Meningiomas are now recognized as the most common brain tumor. They affect the brain around them in different ways depending on their location. They may grow to a great size without producing much problem because the brain squeezes and flattens to accommodate them.

When a person starts to have weakness from the pressure of these tumors, however, the situation becomes critical because brain damage caused by the tumor might be permanent. Increasing symptoms mean the brain can no longer put up with the pressure the tumor produces. Mr. Salvo's tumor had grown to be the size of an orange without many symptoms during its growth. It had reached a critical stage when I first saw him; even a day could make a difference in recovery. This underlay the decision to do surgery the next afternoon.

Surgery. Removal can reverse the meningioma's effect if it is done in time. Unlike gliomas or metastatic tumors, meningiomas just press on the brain rather than infiltrating it; they can be treated by surgery without destroying brain tissue directly. Mr. Salvo's tumor was large and delicately located within the movement area of the brain, making removal an urgent necessity but also a great challenge.

The MRI used to help with surgery not only defines the size and location of the tumor but may be incorporated into surgical navigation. This requires special sequences and post-processing, sequences that were just being "perfected" at the time of Mr. Salvo's surgery. Now they are a routine part of preoperative imaging.

The surgical challenge is that the act of removing the tumor deranges the environment so the brain in that area stops working for a while. If that area is the speech area of the brain, the patient will not speak correctly; if it is the movement area, he or she will not be able to move just because of the release of pressure.

After an operation, the surgeon may not know whether the brain has merely been "stunned" by the surgery or physically damaged. The best test is how long the recovery of function takes. Something as small as movement of a toe may be the sign of significant recovery, as it was for Mr. Salvo.

The recovery of function noted here may seem agonizingly slow to the reader and must have been an eternity for Mr. Salvo. In fact, it is remarkably fast.

Within six weeks of his operation he was walking, which suggests a mild dysfunction of the brain, possibly just the result of manipulating the tumor. The legs are the first to go and the last to improve in tumors in this part of the head.

Steroid psychosis. The swelling that follows any manipulation of brain tissue is best treated by anti-inflammatory medication called corticosteroids. In some patients, these important drugs can have a severe psychological effect—"steroid psychosis." In the rare patient who shows this side effect, the results can be devastating. Managing it is a balance between maintaining some steroids so the brain can heal and avoiding the severe psychological effects.

Radiation. Many people believe that radiation is only used for malignant tumors, but that is less and less true today. Mr. Salvo's tumor was "atypical", an official designation of tumor type. Atypical meningiomas tend to recur more than their typical counterparts, and radiation is an important way of keeping them from recurring.

Dr. Jay Loeffler is one of the pioneers in showing that radiation can slow meningioma recurrence and is also a trailblazer in performing radiation therapy with minimal side effects. The mask Mr. Salvo describes allows very precise radiation to be given just to the tumor bed and not to the surrounding brain. His twenty plus year survival is testimony to the capacity of major surgery and careful radiation to allow recurrence-free life.

Family and friends. Studies on recovery from medical intervention repeatedly demonstrate that a positive social situation facilitates maximum rehabilitation. Mr. Salvo's extensive network of family, friends, and collaborating health professionals created a matrix in which his determination and hard work could thrive.

Faith. As important as his social environment was Mr. Salvo's faith—an unfaltering belief that God would take care of him. The visits of Father Egan, of the parishioners who deluged him with cards and calls, and his own prayers are strong witnesses to the power of this feature of his story.

More can be said than that. Because of a grounding in Christian faith, Mr. Salvo could trust his doctors and his nurses and his caregivers and could work with them for his recovery, convinced he would triumph. Paul says in Philippians 4:13 *"I can do all things through Christ who strengthens me."* Mr. Salvo's story lives that promise.

Determination. Throughout his rehabilitation, Mr. Salvo appeared to have had the single goal of improving his strength and stamina. His description of turning off the TV and lights and truly focusing on the exercises set for him exemplified this dogged determination. When he believed well-wishers were interfering with his physiotherapy, he limited their visits. When a medication dose was wrong, he challenged the nurse. When he felt he could do more than his caregivers allowed, he asked to be allowed to do it. He put his rehabilitation above all other considerations.

As a counterexample, he describes another patient with a similar history who remained wheelchair bound because of lack of effort and negative attitude.

As I read this book again, two observations strike me. The first is the power and mystery of the human brain. Here is an organ that can withstand the pressure of an orange-sized mass in a confined space, then go from non-function to almost full function in two months after major surgery. It can allow full speech and thought in a patient temporarily paralyzed because of its compartmentalization. What a gift it is to be able to work with such a remarkable entity!

The second is that neurosurgery is a team sport. We live in a city where our medical teams are every bit as spectacular as the Red Sox, Patriots, Celtics, Bruins, and others. The surgical resources of hospitals like Brigham and Women's and its nurses, doctors and technicians who make them great medical institutions; the facilities of Wingate and its sister rehabilitation centers; the excellence of radiation oncology for the brain exemplified by people like Jay Loeffler; the outpatient and continuing care capabilities of our region. We are fortunate to live in a city and a country where excellence in medical care is assumed.

Mr. Salvo has kind words for me, but a player is only as good as his or her team. This book is really a tribute to the medical teams of Boston, and it is a dazzling tribute indeed.

Peter Black, M.D., Ph.D., F.A.C.S.
Franc D. Ingraham Professor of Neurosurgery, Emeritus, Harvard Medical School
Founding Chair, Department of Neurosurgery, Brigham and Women's Hospital
February 2019

PREFACE

Recovering from my brain tumor without all the love and support I received before, during, and after surgery would have been extremely difficult, but not unattainable, if I had faced this challenge on my own.

When I left the rehabilitation facility in 1999, the entire medical staff encouraged me to write a book that chronicled my experience. They felt that my journey would give hope to others who had dealt, or were presently dealing, with a life-changing experience. It has taken twenty years to put my thoughts on paper, but I feel like this is the right time because I am currently being monitored for three additional small tumors. What also inspired me was observing others who suffer through various disorders and hardships and don't have the drive to or belief that they can overcome their difficulties.

My misfortune has presented me with the knowledge and opportunity to write a book that could only be written by someone who has been through such hardship. One would have had to *walk in my footsteps* to understand the path I have traveled and the obstacles I have had to overcome. Hopefully, after reading this book, if needed and if the situation is warranted, one will come to the realization that one's objective can indeed be attained after all.

The content of this book and the dialogue contained in it are fully authentic and factual, albeit some of the conversations are not verbatim. Before and after surgery, my dear friend Ann Ormond took precise notes at every doctor's appointment and staff meeting, and that information was placed directly into this book. The notes she compiled at any meeting at Wingate at Brighton as well as a copy of the notes attained from staff members have been included in the text. Lists of medications, including instructions, were transcribed verbatim from the staff.

In my first six days in the hospital, I was extremely aware of what took place, but I also relied on my Mother, my brother Skip, my sister Patty, and Ann for information. I was amazed at the details and conversations I recalled during the writing of this book, because the events described in it occurred twenty-one years ago. It is as if everything I went through during that time was stored in a certain part of my brain, just waiting to be released. During my recovery, my total focus was on walking again; therefore, I thought about nothing else.

When I was released from the hospital and entered the rehabilitation facility, my sister brought in a journal. With my verbal assistance, she transcribed notes of what had taken place in the hospital. Each night in the rehabilitation facility, Ann, my sister, and eventually I would write explicit notes on what had occurred that day. This was of great assistance in the writing of this book, in that some memories were so clear that I was oblivious to everything else around me; indeed, it seemed that I was transported back to the hospital and rehab facility. Upon returning home after my rehabilitation, I continued to keep track of my daily progress.

Some of the daily occurrences may appear to be repetitious, but my intent was to keep my story factual, and in reality, certain statements or actions did keep reoccurring, as was the case with my prayers in the morning and my praying of the Rosary each evening.

Any names appearing in this book have been used with the permission of the individuals. After so many years, I have lost contact with the medical staff at Wingate at Brighton and therefore was unable to list any of them by name.

You will notice that throughout the contents of the book "Mother" and "Father" are capitalized. Although this is not grammatically correct, it was done intentionally to honor my parents for the untold love, inspiration, and support they have given and continue to give me during my lifetime.

INTRODUCTION

I am Joseph C. Salvo, the author of this book, and I would like to thank you for choosing it. Hopefully you have chosen this book simply to read about my journey to overcome adversity, but it was also written for anyone who is confronted with a bump in the road to realize that he or she has the ability to face obstacles head-on and come out on the other side. You can never underestimate the power of the human spirit. If you have the misfortune of a setback, this book will prove that you can achieve any goal you desire.

Since being diagnosed with a brain tumor in 1999, I have had twenty years to contemplate how this could have happened. There were many things I worried about growing up, but this was not one of them. I worried about my Dad, who had a rare vascular disease, Behcet's syndrome, or Behcet's disease,[1] which he contracted traveling from one island to the next in the army during World War II. I worried about when he would inevitably be hospitalized again and how long his stay would be this time. I worried about my Mother being my Father's caregiver and simultaneously raising four children. Then there were the financial issues. Because of his duty in the service, my Father was being seen by doctors in the Veterans Hospital, who believed my Father was having strokes and seizures. The doctors had no reason to assume the strokes and

---

[1] It occurs most frequently in the Middle East and Asia. Turkey has the highest prevalence rate (80 - 370 cases per 100,000); Japan, Korea, China, Iran, and Saudi Arabia also have high prevalence rates. The disorder is the leading cause of blindness in Japan. Ronald R. Butendieck, MD, FACP, Behcet's Syndrome, National Organization for Rare Disorders, raredisease.org

seizures were service related. With the continual deterioration of his health, he was eventually forced to quit work. We never had enough money to maintain a healthy lifestyle until my Father was diagnosed with Behcet's and approved for disability. We then began to receive financial government support. Once he was diagnosed, I invariably feared the disease was hereditary, even after completing some extensive research that indicated it was not.

One thing I never had to worry about was the quality of food we ate. Both sets of grandparents immigrated to the United States from Italy. They grew all their own food and raised chickens and rabbits. They were serving *farm to table* decades before it became a national food trend. What I didn't realize was what I should have been worrying about, where my family was living.

Let's go back to the year 1960. I was eight years old and moving into a new home with the rest of my family: my Mom, Dad, sister, and brother Skip. The house was across the street from a fire station and less than a mile from a couple companies. The companies manufactured many items, such as tubes in radios and microwaves. In the 1960s, there was less awareness of how toxins could alter a person's immune system. Little did I know that the decision of where my parents chose to live, I believe, would change the trajectory of the rest of my life. To add insult to injury, I worked at one of the companies' exit gates selling newspapers. Aside from the number of serious health issues that have plagued, and continue to plague, my former neighborhood, there is no detailed proof of this theory.

Let's jump ahead to 1999 when my nightmare begins. At that time, I was teaching computers to middle schoolers. One day, while at work, I began to experience a weakness on my left side. Within two weeks, I had visited three different doctors, had four MRIs, was diagnosed with a meningioma tumor, and endured twelve hours of *very delicate brain surgery*. Postop I spent a week in the hospital, during which time I experienced a steroid psychosis.[2] From there, I entered a rehabilitation facility where I would live for three and a half weeks. The staff there was kind and compassionate but hinted to me that life as I knew it would be forever changed.

I wouldn't hear of it.

With a daily schedule of grueling physical and occupational therapy and love and support from family, friends, and staff, I was able to get my life back. Though left with some residual effects from the surgery, my recovery has been described by the medical field as "a miracle." You will see that word used several times throughout this book and be amazed at the sequence of events that enabled me to be operated on in a timely manner by a surgeon who was considered to be the best in the world.

In the past twenty years, numerous people have inquired about, and encouraged me to write a book. I felt the time was right because, as mentioned, I am currently being monitored for three small tumors. In May of 2018, the tumors were remaining dormant, but my most recent MRI, on June 18, 2020, detected a very slight increase in size in all three tumors—approximately one-sixth of an inch. The surgeon and I agreed that because there was change, scheduling a yearly MRI for May of 2021 was reasonable. I don't dwell on this situation because of the minimal change. If there is ever major growth in any or all of the tumors, I will make a decision at that time on what should be done. Thanks to radiation performed by Dr. Jay Loeffler, no tumors have developed in the area that was radiated.

My wish for you is that after reading this book, if life presents you with an unimaginable challenge, you will think of me and remember that with determination, hard work, and God's help, anything is possible.

---

[2] *Psychosis* refers to an abnormal condition of the mind described as involving a "loss of contact with reality." People experiencing psychosis may exhibit some personality changes and thought disorder. Depending on its severity, this may be accompanied by unusual or bizarre behavior (Wikipedia, s.v. "psychosis," https://en.wikipedia.org/wiki/Psychosis).

CHAPTER 1
IS THIS THE CAUSE?

As mentioned in the introduction, from my early childhood until his death in 1995, my father's health was poor and continued to decline. He gradually became legally blind and partially paralyzed. He spent weeks, and occasionally months, in the hospital for care and rehabilitation. He was an amazing individual who never complained and constantly said, "I will take whatever God gives me."

When I was fourteen years old, I started working outside a factory near our home selling newspapers. I enjoyed the income and the convenience of the factory being in such close proximity to our home. At the time, my father was still employed, despite his constant hospitalization. The company he worked for was very sympathetic and caring.

While I was working at a gate outside the factory, it was a daily occurrence to observe thick smoke billowing out of the factory smokestacks. During a rainstorm, I assumed chemicals from the smokestacks ended up on the plants in the garden, which we eventually consumed. I never thought of it at the time and never considered it could be harmful. Similar to smoking cigarettes, no one ever realized the consequences until it was too late.

In 1967, my Father had to quit his job because of his declining health. As he needed constant attention, my Mother's primary responsibility was to care for him. With neither parent working and at fifteen years old, I became the sole provider for our family—my parents, my younger sister, my younger brother, and myself. Because of my age, I wasn't old enough to attain working papers, which would have allowed me to work in other establishments. So, I had to continue selling newspapers.

In the winter months, I shoveled snow, and in the spring, I continued selling newspapers and mowed lawns on weekends. That summer, I was old enough to work full-time as a busboy at a restaurant during the week and continued mowing lawns on the weekend. My earnings kept our family afloat. Shortly after I turned sixteen, my father was diagnosed with Behcet's disease and approved for government assistance because they deemed his disability was service related. Finances became less of a burden.

As many times as my father had been in the hospital, I had never been. Once he was diagnosed, I continued to be concerned about the disease being hereditary because I was conceived after he returned from the service. As indicated, I did some research but never found any information to support that assumption.

When growing up, I tried to be very conscious of what I put in my body by eating well, not doing drugs, having only an occasional drink, and not smoking. I never factored in that where I lived would probably be responsible for my future. I believe that once these toxins are free-flowing in your body, they wreak havoc on your future physical development. Everything I did properly didn't prevent the tumor from growing, but it did give me a strong enough body to fight after my surgery.

CHAPTER 2
WHAT'S HAPPENING?

THURSDAY, MARCH 11, 1999

I was in my fifth year of teaching grade six computers in the computer lab at John F. Kennedy Middle School in Waltham, Massachusetts. It was a modern two-story building of bricks and concrete. Waltham is a suburb city about thirteen miles west of Boston. I taught computer applications, such as the internet, Microsoft Word, Excel, PowerPoint, Access, and Publisher. I also taught business applications—for instance, how to type a professional business letter and envelopes. Besides my grade six classes, other disciplines would sign up for the computer lab and bring their students into the class. They would teach their subject area, and I would teach the computer aspect of the subject.

It was about ten in the morning, and I was walking down the hall, which was well lit because of the numerous windows. Yet suddenly, I took a misstep with my left leg and almost fell. I looked down to see if there was a rug or any object on the floor that may have caused my near fall. Not noticing anything, I thought it was strange because I was pretty sure-footed, but I dismissed it as just a misstep and continued to walk without incident. Although I didn't realize it at the time, this was my first sign of a problem. I finished the school day without giving it another thought.

Around four in the afternoon, I went home to my apartment, an apartment I rented in my Parent's house in Waltham. After dinner, I corrected some papers, watched some TV, and went to bed around ten, because tomorrow was another school day.

FRIDAY, MARCH 12

The next morning was the same as any other. I got up, ate breakfast, showered, shaved, and headed off for my ten-minute drive to school. During the day, I needed some supplies from the top shelf of the closet and reached up with both arms. My left arm was very weak. I wasn't in a lot of pain, but it felt as if someone were squeezing my arm. I assumed I had pulled a muscle, and it would go away. I finished the rest of the day without any problem with my leg, but my left arm continued to feel weak whenever I raised it above my shoulder. I still wasn't overly concerned, so being Friday, after school, I headed to my home in Mashpee, on Cape Cod, Massachusetts, where I spent vacations, holidays, and weekends.

The hour-and-a-half drive took me away from the hustle and bustle of Waltham. Waltham had a historically industrial base, including making Waltham Watches, but now it had many high-tech businesses, a population of sixty thousand, and a lot of traffic. Mashpee had a population of fourteen thousand, forests and preserves, and numerous beaches on Vineyard Sound, which overlooked the island of Martha's Vineyard off in the distance.

SATURDAY AND SUNDAY, MARCH 13 AND 14

Over the weekend, I had no problems walking, but anytime I tried to reach above my shoulder, my left arm continued to feel weak. I again assumed it was just a pulled muscle and dismissed it as such.

MONDAY, MARCH 15

Monday morning, I drove back to school from the Cape. The traffic became heavier the closer I got to Boston and the businesses along Route 95 in Waltham.

During the middle of the day, I was walking up the stairs at school and took another misstep with my left foot. I fell on my knees. Now I began to worry that there was definitely something wrong. I continued the day without another incident but called my primary-care doctor after school and told his nurse what had happened. She said she would explain the situation to the doctor and have him call me back. I gave her the school number, and he called back in half an hour.

He said he obviously couldn't diagnose the problem over the phone but would like to see me the following day. He said he would have the nurse set up an appointment and transferred the call. I didn't want to miss any school, so I told her I could come immediately after school around three thirty; she agreed and set up the appointment. It was good of them to get me in on such short notice. I was concerned but never thought it was anything catastrophic. I, once again, continued the day as if nothing had happened. I knew that I would get an explanation for what was happening the next day.

TUESDAY, MARCH 16

The next morning between home and school, the missteps became more frequent. My left arm was still very weak. I hadn't told anyone and became more concerned, because the problems were getting increasingly worse. My mind started wondering about what could possibly be wrong. *Do I have a blood clot? Do I have a disease? Could it be Behcet's, even though everything I have read said it is not hereditary?* Hopefully, I would have more information that afternoon after visiting my primary-care doctor. I left immediately after school and drove to the appointment.

5

I arrived at the medical building around 3:15. I knew the doctor was somewhat concerned because he told the nurse to tell me to come in immediately after school, and he would see me as soon as I arrived. I checked in and sat down in the waiting room for about three minutes before the nurse came to get me and walked me into the exam room. She took all my vitals. My pulse and temperature were perfect, but, not surprisingly, my blood pressure was elevated, as I assumed it might be. The doctor entered a few minutes later and asked me to describe what had been taking place over the last few days. I told him about the missteps and that they were becoming more frequent, and I also talked about the weakness in my left arm.

He gave me a complete physical and then asked me to put my hands together out in front of my body as if I were praying. Once I did this, he placed both his hands outside of mine and asked me to push outward as hard as I could. I had no problem with my right hand but could barely move my left. He then asked me to put both my arms shoulder height straight in front of my body. He placed his hands inside of mine and asked me to push in as hard as possible. Same results—no problem with my right hand but weakness with the left. He then asked me to sit on the table with my legs out straight. He placed one hand outside each leg and asked me to push outward. My legs had the same results as my arms, strong with the right but very weak with the left. He then asked me to bring my legs to the same position, and he put his hands on the inside and asked me to push inward against his resistance. My right leg was very strong, but my left leg would barely move.

He excused himself and left the office. Now I was alone to contemplate what the tests meant. When he returned, he said he wasn't sure what was happening, but I definitely needed to have an MRI.

I said, "What's an MRI?"

He explained that an MRI, or a magnetic resonance imaging scan, is a common scan that uses a strong magnetic field and radio waves to create detailed images of the organs and tissues within the body. He explained that I would be placed on a table that slid into a tube, and the machine would take images of the inside of my body. I asked him if he had any idea of what was going on. He said he wasn't sure, but an MRI would give a clearer picture. I asked where I would set up an appointment. He said he already had; it was the following morning at 8:30. I was to see the nurse before I left, and she would give me directions to the MRI center. I thanked him and left the office. I visited with the nurse, collected my paperwork and directions, and headed home.

I drove home and, on the way, realized there had to be something serious going on for him to order an MRI first thing the next morning. Once again, I began to wonder what it could possibly be. I still considered that it might be Behcet's, even though the medical books stated it was not hereditary and the symptoms were different than my Father's. Could it be a blood clot? But how could a blood clot affect both my left leg and left arm at the same time? If it was, could it be dissolved? Would I end up in the hospital and if so for how long? I couldn't miss school, even though I had three hundred sick days. Hopefully it was not as serious as I was imagining and just something minor. If that were the case, why would the doctor order an MRI for the next morning? Maybe he was not sure, and just wanted to be proactive. All of these thoughts, and more, were circulating around in my head, which was spinning.

I had to tell my Mother something but what? She would worry no matter what I said, so I had to phrase my words so she wouldn't panic. When I arrived home, I told her I had a weakness in my left arm and decided to see the doctor to make sure there was nothing wrong. I told her he wasn't sure what the problem was, if any, but I would be having an MRI the next day to find out what was going on. Of course, she had a hundred questions. I said that we would have more answers the following day. I went upstairs to my apartment to correct some of my students' papers that I had brought home with me. That afternoon, I called the substitute service for the next day.

I went to bed early that night but didn't sleep very well. I was more anxious than nervous to find out what was happening.

WEDNESDAY, MARCH 17

The next morning, I arrived early at school and went to my computer lab to leave some instructions for the substitute. I then went to the main office to tell the administration that I was going to be out for the day and that I had left instructions for the substitute. I explained my circumstance and told them I would be leaving to have an MRI. On my way out of the office, the secretary said her computer wasn't working correctly and asked if I could fix it. I told her I was heading out for a doctor's appointment and would come back and take a look at it that afternoon. She said it would probably only take a couple of minutes, and I said my doctor had ordered an MRI and I was on my way there. She said she understood and would do her best to get her work done without it. Even though I was a computer teacher and not a technician, they still relied heavily on my ability to troubleshoot their computers when they had a problem.

I decided to drive alone to the MRI to prevent anyone from needlessly worrying about me. During the ride, my thoughts were all over the place about what this could be. Could it be nerve damage, or did I injure myself? I didn't remember doing anything that would affect my leg and arm. I arrived at the center and walked into a bright office with a few chairs, some pictures on the wall, and magazines on a table. I introduced myself to the secretary, who was seated behind a sliding glass window and gave her the paperwork from the doctor's office.

She said, "Please be seated and fill out this paperwork, and the technician will be with you shortly."

I filled out three sheets of questions about my health and then returned the completed forms to the secretary.

I sat down and started to read a magazine. About fifteen minutes later, the technician, a short and very thin individual, came into the waiting area. In a soft-spoken voice, he introduced himself and asked me to follow him. He retrieved the paperwork I had left with the secretary and then took me into a small office.

"Everything looks fine," he said. "There should be no problems with the MRI." He asked a few questions, and the last question was if I had ever had an MRI.

I said, "I don't want to appear ignorant, but I not only haven't had one, but I have no idea what it is."

He said, "It stands for magnetic resonance imaging. It's a machine. I will show it to you shortly, and it will scan your body. Because it works off magnets, you have to remove all metal from your body."

He told me to follow him into the changing room. He said, "Anything metal must be removed and placed into this locker, and then remove the key and put it on the shelf in the scan room."

I removed all my metal, including my belt, keys, and change in my pocket and placed them into the locker.

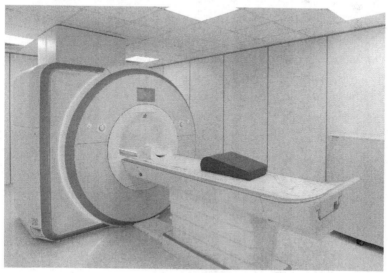

Magnetic resonance imaging machine.

I asked if I had to remove my Crucifix and chain, which my grandmother had given me in 1960 and had been part of me and never taken off for thirty-nine years.

He was very nice and explained that any metal would alter the results, so it couldn't be worn. I removed my Crucifix and chain, kissed it, placed it into the locker, closed the door, and removed the key. This was very traumatic because not only did I consider myself fairly religious but this Crucifix was given to me by my grandmother, and wearing it gave me a sense of comfort and security. I felt as if part of me had been detached; no matter what, it had to be removed.

As it was my first MRI, I didn't fully understand what he was talking about with regards to removing all my metal. He explained it, but my brain was still in a fog because of what had taken place the last few days.

I followed him into a dimly lit room that contained a huge tube. It was about eight feet long and about three feet wide and situated a few feet off the floor. Extending from this tube was a table approximately the same size upon which I assumed I would lie before being placed into the MRI tube.

He said, "You will lie on the table, and then we will place a helmet over your head for stability. The helmet has a little mirror on it, which is angled so you can see out of the tube. There's nothing to look at, but some people feel more comfortable having it. We will then electronically roll your entire body into the MRI tube for a total of a little over an hour. The machine will produce extremely loud noises and clanging while taking the images, so we suggest you use a set of earplugs to wear. Within the hour, there are various scans that will last two to five minutes, with a short break in between. We will talk to you between each set to see how you're doing. During this entire MRI, you need to remain as still as possible. If the scan doesn't come out clear, we have to repeat the procedure. Any questions?"

"I am claustrophobic, so what happens if I panic?"

"Oh yes, I forgot. There's a rubber bulb you can use if you're having a difficult time; just squeeze the bulb, and we'll come in and take you out."

As he was describing this entire procedure, I began contemplating how all of this could have happened in such a short period of time. Just a few days ago, I was smiling and enjoying life, but now I had to undergo this traumatic experience and face an unknown future.

A nurse entered the room, and I told them I was ready, so they placed me on the table, put the helmet over my head from the top down, and then placed the bulb in my right hand. They asked if I was comfortable, and I said, "About as comfortable as I can be."

They said, "All right, here we go."

They pushed the button that rolled me into the MRI, which left me with about five inches from my nose to the top of the tube. The mirror allowed me to see out of the tube, but I was still nervous. I could see the MRI technician setting up the scan in a room on the other side of the glass. He could speak to me through an intercom and asked if I was doing okay. I said yes. The only reason I didn't press the bulb was because I realized this was something that had to be done; I had to struggle through all the banging and clanging. I was indeed feeling claustrophobic but knew I had no other options. Completing this MRI was essential because without it, there would be no answers to why I was having these problems. Knowing that, I stayed perfectly still during each scan but would still hyperventilate during the short breaks while he set up the next scan.

Without the little mirror on my helmet, I am not sure I could have mentally endured the entire hour. I constantly thought about what would happen if we lost power. Would they be able to get me out because my helmet was put on from the top down, and I only had about five inches to the top of the tube? With the tube being a specific size, I also wondered how overweight people fit inside. Through all the banging and clanging, one's mind continues to wander and question what's taking place. It is often said that "time flies," but in this machine, that hour seemed like forever. Once the

11

MRI was complete, they told me they were on their way, and then came in and flicked the switch to roll me out. They took the helmet off and told me to slowly stand up from the table, which I did.

I said, "Thank You, God."

They then walked me back to my locker, and I put all my belongings back on. The assistant guided me to a private office and told me to take a seat and the radiologist would read the scan and come in to speak with me. There was nothing in the room except a few chairs and a wall monitor to display the scan. I waited for about twenty minutes, and the radiologist finally arrived. He asked how I had done with the MRI. I said, "It wasn't very comfortable, and I hope I never have to go through anything like that again. What did the scan show?"

He said, "I will show you on the monitor."

He took the x-ray of the scan and placed it on the wall monitor and then turned it on. He spoke very calmly, as if he were telling me I had a cavity in one of my teeth.

"This is your scan, and this large mass outside your brain is a meningioma tumor. It's very large and must be removed very soon."

I said, "How is that done? Can it be drained? Can it be dissolved? How are we going to remove it?"

I was anxious and asking multiple questions even before he answered my first one. I really had no idea what had to be done, and I think I was in a state of shock.

He said, "No, you have to have *major, major* surgery."

It's strange because through all of this there are some statements I remember verbatim like "major, major."

I said, "This is terrible news."

He said, "I am fairly certain that it's benign and can be removed without a problem, but it will have to be removed very soon."

I said, "That is still terrible news."

He said, "Joe, there are some patients with a tumor, and I am pretty sure it's malignant. All I tell them is that they have a tumor and will have to see a neurosurgeon for a more thorough exam. The good news is I have a doctor who is phenomenal and I believe to be the best in the world, and he works in Boston, Dr. Peter Black."

He went on to praise him and stated he was the neurosurgeon in chief of three major hospitals in Boston. He continued to glorify him for approximately fifteen minutes and said, "Let me give his office a call and set up an appointment."

I said, "I have to sit down." The news to him wasn't devastating, but all I could think of was his saying, "*major, major* surgery."

He left, went into his office, and called Brigham and Women's Hospital and spoke to the secretary. I could hear him asking for an appointment with Dr. Black, and after twenty seconds, his response was a loud "*What!*" I knew something was wrong.

He returned and said, "Unfortunately, Dr. Black is out of the country and won't be back anytime soon. But don't worry; I have another doctor who is pretty good."

As I said before, there are some statements that I will never forget. I raised my voice. "You told me I have to have *major, major* surgery, and I am getting *pretty good.*"

I think he was so stunned that Dr. Black wasn't available he wasn't aware of what he was saying and just blurted it out. He apologized and said, "I am sorry. I should have said, 'Excellent.'"

I said, "But you didn't; you said, 'Pretty good.'"

He left the room and called the doctor's office. He explained that I had to be seen immediately and set up an appointment for the next day. I thanked him and left the office.

I was more in shock than concerned. I wasn't scared but a little nervous, not knowing what was about to happen in the near future. On the ride home, I prayed a Rosary and told God that I was putting it in His hands. I also thought of my Mother, who was home waiting for me. It took about forty minutes to get home.

My Mother is a very strong woman. She had endured a lot taking care of my Father for about thirty-five years with thousands of trips to the hospital, cooking him special meals, and taking care of his personal needs at home. As strong as she was through all of his health issues, receiving news that I had a brain tumor would not be pleasant, but I never contemplated how devastating it would be for her. Once home, I knew my Mother would immediately want to know the results of the MRI, so I walked into my Mother's home while she was cleaning the outside of the refrigerator.

She turned to me and nervously asked, "What did the doctor say?"

Not thinking how traumatic the news would be, I told her the doctor said I have a very large brain tumor. Her knees gave out, and she fell against the refrigerator and held onto the handle to keep from falling to the ground. She then started crying hysterically, so I rushed over with a chair. I said, "Please, sit down." I had been fine until this point and then started to apologize. I said I was sorry and that I didn't mean to get a brain tumor. I was so worried about her that I didn't know what to say or do. I said the radiologist said I would have surgery, and everything would be fine. I was just trying to calm her down. (Telling her I had a brain tumor was bad enough, but I remember saying "very large," which was not very bright on my part; I just reiterated what the radiologist had told me.)

I called my younger brother Skip, and he said, "What's wrong? I hear someone crying."

I told him I had a brain tumor, and Mom was hysterical. He said he would be right over. I then called my aunt, my Mother's sister and best friend, and told her the news, and she said she also would be right over. I was trying to console my Mother, and in about ten minutes, my brother showed up.

He said, "What did the doctor say?"

I told him, "He said I have a very large brain tumor, and it will have to be surgically removed sooner rather than later." Looking back, yet again, I should have left out the phrase "very large."

A few minutes later, my aunt arrived, and I repeated the same story to her. All this time, my Mother was sobbing and now being consoled by my brother and aunt. All she kept saying was, "Everything we have been through, and now this. I think we have had enough in our lives. Why is God giving us something else?"

She was talking about my Father and the years of taking care of him twenty-four/seven for most of his life. I think to her, having a brain tumor meant certain death. I should have called my brother and aunt before I came home to have them meet me there. I was in a state of shock and never thought about it.

My brother and aunt stayed for about another hour, and my Mother started to calm down. I told them I had to meet with a surgeon the next day. They both said if I needed company, they would join me. I said I would like to call Ann and see if she could come because she worked in the medical field. She would be able to ask pertinent questions that I would never think of. They agreed and said if she couldn't go, they would join me because I shouldn't go alone. I thanked them and they left. My Mother was still crying, and I told her everything would be fine. I said it was out of our hands, and she agreed. I kissed her and told her I was going up to my apartment to take a nap but would be back before I went to bed for the night. She said she would call my sister, Patty, and brother Chris.

I slowly walked up the steps and tripped on the way, confirming that I had no alternative but to have the tumor removed. I immediately called the school to give them the results and told them I would be out for at least the next couple of days and would call them Friday to let them know the status of my situation. I called the substitute service and told them I would need a substitute for the next two days. Once I got off the phone, I collapsed into the chair. I was exhausted and my head was spinning. I fell asleep in the chair and slept for about an hour before waking up to the ringing of the phone.

I answered the phone, and it was my sister, Patty. She said, "I have been calling you, and no one answered. I called Mom, and she told me you were taking a nap. You never take a nap, so you must be tired."

I told her I was more mentally than physically drained. I explained the whole story, and she said she would be there for me and keep me in her prayers. That was very special because we are only two years apart and very close. She also had health problems at that time; she had been struggling with fibromyalgia for over twenty years. I called a few friends and told them the news. I would hang up, and within minutes, the phone would ring again. It was relatives and friends calling to tell me they had heard the news. My brother Chris called, and I explained everything to him. The phone continued to ring for the next couple of hours. When they say bad news travels fast, they're not kidding. I have no idea how some of these friends even heard, and I didn't ask.

That night, I called Ann Ormond and explained everything. I asked if she would join me the next day for my neurosurgeon's appointment.

She said, "Absolutely. I will meet you at your Mother's at 11:00 a.m. tomorrow."

I felt more at ease knowing Ann would accompany me because she was the Director of Marketing and Community and Public Relations at Waltham Hospital, and as I referenced earlier, she was familiar with the medical field and all the technical jargon.

Before going to bed, I went downstairs to check on my Mother. She had settled down somewhat but was still in tears. I told her everything would be fine, but if God wanted me, He would take me, and we had no say in the matter. I said I would fight through surgery and recovery with everything I had. I then gave her a kiss good night, went up to my own apartment, said some extra-long prayers, and then went to bed.

CHAPTER 3
MEETING DR. "PRETTY GOOD"

THURSDAY, MARCH 18

I actually slept very well and woke up around five thirty as usual. I said my prayers, which I did every morning, ate breakfast, showered, shaved, and then dressed for the day. At 7:15 a.m., I started to receive phone calls from friends and now coworkers who had found out about my condition. I explained the story about my weakness and then told them about the results of the MRI. They all said basically the same thing, that they would keep me in their prayers, if there was anything I needed to please call, and to keep them updated. I no sooner answered one call and the phone would ring again until 10:45 a.m., when I had to start heading downstairs.

I found my Mother still upset, and she said, "I hope everything goes well today."

I said, "I am sure it will."

Ann showed up about five minutes later, so we headed out around 11:00 a.m. to the neurosurgeon who was "pretty good." I was distracted and not in a good place emotionally, so Ann agreed to drive to one of the major hospitals in Boston—I don't remember which hospital. We arrived in the parking garage around 11:45 a.m. We took the elevator and located the doctor's office. We walked into a very bright waiting room with about six chairs and a secretary behind the desk. I went up and introduced myself. I said I had an appointment with the doctor. She asked me to fill out a few forms, and after filling them out, I gave them back to her. She looked them over and said, "The doctor will see you soon."

About fifteen minutes later, a nurse came out and asked Ann and me to follow her. We went into a small office with a table, a few chairs, and a wall monitor.

We sat there for a few minutes, and then the neurosurgeon, who was of average height and weight, entered the office with another doctor, whom he introduced as an assistant in training. We stood up, introduced ourselves, and sat down. The neurosurgeon said he had reviewed the scan, and the tumor was very large. Thankfully, Ann was taking notes, because I was still numb from everything that had happened the day before. He explained that the tumor was a meningioma, which is a slow-growing tumor that grows from the covering of the brain and has a broad base attachment to the falx. It had been there for a number of years and was a little over five centimeters in size, which was a fairly large tumor. They grow at an average of two to three millimeters a year. He said because of its size, there were no other options open to me other than surgery, and the sooner this happened, the better. I am not sure if I didn't hear, or didn't want to hear, what he said, so I asked if it could be dissolved. He said it was too big and had to be removed surgically. He said the tumor was close to the motor strip, the vascular veins, and a major draining vein. It had expanded and pushed into the brain, which was causing pressure and thus the weakness on my left side.

He started to explain the procedure and said it would be done under general anesthesia and would take approximately three to five hours. He would make an incision, elevate the bone temporarily, and micro surgically remove the tumor, being careful of the motor strip. He said it would be a complete excision, and it was a safe operation, but it was still the brain. There would be a potential for seizures, but the likelihood was small. I would be on Dilantin, which would reduce the chance of having a seizure. If he operated on a Monday, I would be home by Friday. It would take six weeks to recuperate but longer to feel 100 percent. A possible side effect would be speech problems, because the left side of my mouth would be weakened. He also said that I would probably have temporary leg weakness until I strengthened it with physical therapy. Pending the outcome of the surgery, there was a 2 to 3 percent chance of needing radiation. I would have to follow up with an MRI each year for five years, but it was unlikely it would reoccur. He asked if we had any questions, but we said we didn't so at that time. We needed time to process all the information and would get back to him in a couple of days.

A great deal of the medical information was beyond my comprehension, but I was hoping Ann would understand and be able to explain it to me. I am thankful Ann took notes verbatim and would explain what was said because to me everything was a blur. It would have been impossible for me to remember this information for this book.

We were there for about an hour, and my head was spinning. He said, "No matter what you decide, you will need to have two more MRIs."

I said I would call my primary-care doctor and set them up.

We left the office and headed back to the car. Once inside the car, I said to Ann, "What do you think?"

She said, "He seems to be well versed about what has to be done and has enough pertinent information, but I don't feel comfortable enough to have him operate on your brain."

"My sentiments exactly. I have to go home and consider my options, because, as the radiologist and neurosurgeon both said, I don't have a lot of time to decide. It's as if he was a computer spitting out information. He didn't seem to show compassion when telling us the protocol. It's just a job."

Ann said, "Exactly."

We both agreed that I should definitely get a second opinion and compare the results, because this was "major, major surgery." I said we shouldn't mention this to my Mother in case Dr. "Pretty Good" was the one who ended up performing the operation.

When we arrived home, Ann and I sat down with my Mother to explain the situation. I did mention he appeared to know exactly what he was talking about, but I never mentioned that we weren't totally comfortable with his performing the surgery. All I said was that it was an operation on my brain, so I still wanted to get a second opinion. Ann said the meeting was very intense—lots of questions and lots of notes. The less I said to my Mother, the better, since she was still in tears from the day before. Ann and I went up to my apartment and had a glass of wine. I said, "What do you think?"

She replied, "Why don't you call Brigham and Women's and tell them you would like a second opinion?"

"That sounds good. I will call you after I speak to them."

I thanked her for all her help, and she left. I thought to myself that the only thing that was clear from this appointment was that I needed surgery; aside from that, the medical jargon was all "Greek to me." I called my primary-care doctor and set up an appointment for two more MRIs. I was so drained and didn't feel up to talking to anyone, so I just lay down and fell asleep. While I was sleeping, the nurse from my doctor's office called and left a message that I had been set up for two more MRIs—one the next day and one on Sunday. I had a few more phone calls inquiring about how my appointment went, and then I said my prayers, lay down, and fell asleep for the night.

FRIDAY, MARCH 19

The next morning, I drove myself into Brigham and Women's at 9:00 a.m. for a second MRI. I am glad I had my first MRI and knew what to expect because this technician was either having a very bad day or shouldn't have been working in patient care. He was about six foot three, 250 pounds, and said with a forceful and stern voice, "This MRI will take one hour and ten minutes, and if you move more than an inch during the process, we'll have to start the entire MRI over." Luckily, everything went well, and I didn't move; actually, I think I was too frightened to move.

On the drive home, I had a light-bulb moment. Why don't I call Kathy Mulcahey, a friend of mine who had a tumor removed in 1998, to find out whom she had for a neurosurgeon? When I arrived home, I immediately called and asked her who her neurosurgeon was. She said, "I had the best in the world: Dr. Peter Black."

I said, "My MRI radiologist raved about him for fifteen minutes, and he actually made the same statement as you, stating he was indeed the best in the world. Unfortunately, as of two days ago, he is out of the country and won't be back for some time."

She said, "No, he came back."

I said, "What do you mean, he's back? How do you know?"

She said, "I just called his office this morning for a follow-up appointment, and they said he had come back to perform emergency surgery on one of his former patients."

"Talk about timing; this is unbelievable. Thank you, Kathy, for that great news. Let me call his office, and hopefully, I can make an appointment to see him."

As soon as I finished my conversation with her, I called his office, and fortunately, he had an opening the following Tuesday, March 23, at 9:00 a.m., so I booked it.

I walked downstairs after booking the appointment and explained to my Mother that everyone said Dr. Black was the best in the world. He was the doctor I wanted to see initially, but he was out of the country and miraculously had just returned. I never mentioned that before because she was upset enough and knowing I wouldn't be able to see him would have only made it worse. I immediately called Ann, told her the news, and asked if she would join me. She said she would love to go, if for nothing else than to have the opportunity to meet the world-renowned Dr. Black. I said, "Once we see him and hear what he has to say, we'll make a well-informed decision. Hopefully, we won't have to make another appointment with any other Dr. 'Pretty Goods.'"

I called the school to tell them that I would be out for an extended period of time. I then called the sub service to inform them I would need a sub for at least two weeks and would call them in a couple of weeks to update them on my progress.

Little did I know, at that time, I would be out of school for the rest of the year. I spent the rest of the day answering phone calls from friends, relatives, and coworkers. I repeatedly told the same story about being able to see Dr. Black. I should have recorded it and played it for each caller. I went to bed early and slept much better.

SATURDAY, MARCH 20

I spent most of the day just hanging around the house, pondering what my future would hold. At this point, I was talking to myself and asking myself hundreds of questions. I felt much better about the situation than I had two days earlier. The phone calls were still coming in. I spent some time with my Mother, who also felt a little better knowing I would be seeing Dr. Black.

I had a relaxing afternoon, then my Mother, Ann, and I went over to my brother Skip's for dinner. After spending a few hours there, I came home, watched a little television, and went to bed.

CHAPTER 4
MEETING DR. PETER BLACK

SUNDAY, MARCH 21

I had my third, and what I thought would be my final, pre-op MRI at 9:00 a.m. Everything was falling into place. Dr. Black had returned, and I was able to book an appointment with him the following Tuesday. I felt so much better now that I had an appointment with Dr. Black. I said to myself, "God is watching over me."

I went to twelve o'clock Mass and then spent the rest of the day hanging around the house, yet again, contemplating what my future would hold and thankful that I didn't have to worry about finding another doctor. A number of family, friends, and coworkers I hadn't spoken to on Saturday left messages inquiring about my appointment with my original surgeon, so I had to return a few more calls. In the afternoon, I had Sunday dinner with my Mother (probably pasta) and then went back upstairs and watched some television. After a few hours, I went to bed and slept better than I had in a week.

MONDAY, MARCH 22

I woke up around 5:30 a.m. as usual and performed my morning routine. I went downstairs to spend some time with my Mother and sister. We went out for a more relaxing lunch. It was a good day, and I believe they were relieved knowing I would be seeing a world-renowned neurosurgeon. We spent about six hours together, and then my sister went home, and I went up to my apartment and slept well that night.

TUESDAY, MARCH 23

I woke up much happier knowing I would be seeing Dr. Black that day. I did my morning routine and then headed downstairs around 7:00 a.m. Ann arrived at 7:15, and we headed into Brigham and Women's at 7:30 a.m. for a 9:00 a.m. appointment. We wanted to make sure we were there on time. We arrived early and parked in the parking garage and then made our way to his office. We entered a very large office, which I would later learn was

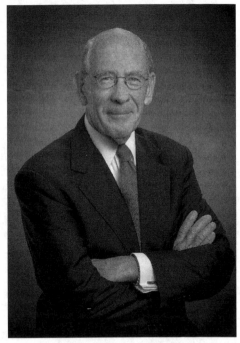

Peter Black, M.D., Ph.D., F.A.C.S.

shared with other doctors. I introduced myself to the secretary and stated that I had an appointment with Dr. Black.

She asked me to fill out some paperwork, which contained questions very similar to the ones asked by Dr. "Pretty Good." I kept quiet and filled them out, thinking to myself there must be a way for them to share this information. I gave the secretary the paperwork, and she said, "Please have a seat; the nurse will inform you when it's time."

Donna DelloIacono came out at 9:45 a.m., introduced herself as Dr. Black's nurse, and brought us into his office. As Ann and I entered, this stately gentleman in a white coat who was sitting alone in his office stood up and introduced himself. Ann and I introduced ourselves, and I noticed his handshake was very stern but soft; my immediate thought was, *Great hands for a surgeon.* He was of average height and build, wore glasses, and had salt-and-pepper hair. In a very soft voice, his first statement was, "I want you to be aware of what will take place, so once I am done explaining … *if you need ten minutes, I will give you ten minutes; if you need three hours, I will give you three hours.* I want you to be very comfortable before going into surgery and have all your questions answered."

As previously mentioned, there are some statements I never forgot, and this was one. Not hearing another word, Ann and I looked at each other with a smile knowing this was definitely the doctor who should be, and would be, operating on me.

He said that he had read the scan and that it was a very large meningioma tumor. He estimated it had been growing for approximately ten years, and surgery was my only option. I would be administered general anesthesia or could remain awake for the operation, which would take roughly six to eight hours. There would be a slight chance of seizures, but I would be on Dilantin, which is a seizure medication. There would be weakness on the left side because of the position of the brain. I would need physical therapy to strengthen my leg and arm. There would be a 5 percent chance of radiation and a 1 percent chance of a steroid psychosis. Dr. Black reiterated most of what "Dr. Pretty Good" had told us, with some subtle changes. He legally had to mention some of the potential severe consequences of surgery. Convinced that he would perform the surgery, Ann didn't take as many notes. He asked us if we had any questions.

I said, "No, we would like you to perform the surgery."

"Don't the both of you want to discuss it?"

"We already have with our smiles to each other."

He said, "Unfortunately, there could be a potential problem." I think I stopped breathing for at least ten seconds. "The tumor must be removed immediately, so prior to this meeting, I checked, and there are no operating rooms available in the near future ... Hold on, and let me recheck."

When he left, Ann and I both agreed that if a room was available, this was the doctor we wanted to perform the surgery. I remember praying and asking God to please let there be a room open.

Dr. Black came back about ten minutes later and said, "It's amazing, but in that short period of time, there has been a cancellation and an operating room is available."

Before he even finished his statement, I said, "We'll take it."

He said, "It's at 4:00 p.m. tomorrow. Would the two of you first like to discuss it before you decide?"

I said, "We already did while you were gone."

Even though Ann and I had only known him for forty-five minutes, he made us feel so comfortable; it was as if we had known him for some time. We felt confident about him performing the operation.

He said, "That works out well because I am actually performing another surgery prior to yours. Do you have any other questions for me?"

"What does the operation actually entail?" I asked.

"Would you prefer to be awake for the operation or under anesthesia?"

"Definitely under anesthesia, because I don't want to hear what's going on."

"Then first we'll set up an IV and put you under. Then I will mark your head where I will make the cut. Then with the saw—"

"Okay, I think I heard enough."

He said, "Any other questions?"

"This may be a foolish question, but never having been through anything like this before, how many of your patients have not made it through the operation?"

He looked at me and said, *"All of my patients have made it through."*

"That makes me feel so much better. I think that's all I have for questions." I asked Ann if she had any questions, and she said no.

He said, "So I will see you tomorrow at 4:00 p.m. sharp."

On our way out, Ann and I shook his hand, and as I was walking out the door, I said, "Now be on your best behavior tonight so you'll be in good form tomorrow, because *my life is in your hands and God's hands.*"

"Absolutely," he replied.

I closed the door, walked about five feet, thought about that statement, turned around, opened the door, and said, "But not in that order."

"I totally agree," he said.

On the ride home, I said to Ann, "We only spoke with him for about an hour, but I can't imagine anyone else operating on me except Dr. Black. I see why he has the reputation he does. His overall demeanor is far superior to Dr. Pretty Good's. The way he talks to you and instills the fact that you are in great hands and everything will be fine."

Ann totally agreed.

We went home and explained to my Mother about all that had transpired on our visit, informing her of what a wonderful doctor he was and that his mannerisms were of such high quality.

Ann said, "He is very patient, kind, and caring. We are unwavering in our faith in him and his abilities."

My Mother asked, "Did you make an appointment for surgery?"

I said, "We did; it's tomorrow at 4:00 p.m."

She blurted out very loudly, "*What? Tomorrow?* Why so soon? Couldn't you have waited a while?"

"Dr. Black said it must be removed immediately, and tomorrow was the only time an operating room was available. I don't want to wait; what would I wait for? I want to get this over with as soon as possible."

"Let me call your brothers and sister and give them the news."

Ann said, "I have to get going," so I thanked her for all she had done.

"Will I see you tomorrow?" I asked.

"Absolutely."

"Great," I said and then went up to my apartment.

It was a whirlwind of a day, and I wanted to lie down, but of course, the phone was ringing off the hook. My Mother got the word out, and the calls were coming in. First, my sister called, and I spoke to her for a little while, until my doorbell rang; it was my brother Skip, who was at the bottom of the stairs. When I opened the door, all he said was a louder-than-normal "*Tomorrow?*"

"Yes," I said. "That's the only time an operating room was available, and I want to get this over with."

Two minutes later, my brother Chris called, and I filled him in on what was happening the following day. As soon as I got off the phone with Chris, the phone rang. Skip yelled up, "Let me go, and I will call you tonight and drive you in tomorrow."

For the next couple of hours, the phone rang constantly, and I continued to tell the same story. My brother Skip eventually called and said he would pick me up at two thirty the next day to take me to the hospital.

I went to bed at eight, hoping to get a good night's sleep, and around nine, the phone rang again, but this time the call was from Brigham and Women's Hospital, informing me I had to come to the hospital that night to have another MRI.

I said, "They told me I only had to have three."

She said, "They actually perfected a three-dimensional MRI earlier today, which is better than the other three combined. You must be praying because the timing of this is amazing considering you will be operated on tomorrow. It will be very instrumental in helping Dr. Black with the surgery."

I said, "I have been saying a considerable amount of prayers."

I got out of bed, got dressed, called my Mother to explain the situation, and then called Skip to ask him if he would drive me into Brigham and Women's. He said that would not be a problem. On the way to the hospital, I thought to myself that I couldn't believe the timing of the events of the past few days:

I called Kathy Mulcahey, who out of hundreds of surgeons in Boston had Dr. Black, whom I originally wanted to see and who was now back in Boston.

Dr. Black had an opening in his schedule to see me.

An operating room became available.

Just that day, the day before my surgery, they perfected a three-dimensional MRI, better than any they had had in the past.

Someone was definitely looking after me. I prayed a Rosary to thank God for His divine intervention the past few days and asked for His blessings for a successful surgery the next day. I made it to the hospital, had the MRI, went home, and went to bed.

CHAPTER 5
THE OPERATION

WEDNESDAY, MARCH 24

I woke up around 5:30 a.m. and was surprised at how well I had slept. I said my prayers, took a shower, shaved, and watched a little television, for the weather report. It was an overcast day with temperatures ranging from the mid-thirties to mid-fifties. I wanted to make sure I dressed appropriately; I couldn't afford to become sick. I hung around the house for a while and received about a dozen phone calls. Each one ended by wishing me well and offering prayers for a successful surgery.

At 9:00 a.m., I walked downstairs to my Mother's. She was still nervous and asked me how I had slept. I told her I had slept really well and was at peace with whatever happened that day because it was now in God's hands. She agreed but said she had only slept about two hours. I understood her anxiety; facing the unknown is always daunting. *Even I had no knowledge as to what would take place the next month.*

I stayed downstairs for about an hour and then walked back up to my apartment. I prayed a Rosary a few times before getting ready to leave for the hospital. I had to be there by 4:00 p.m., so we had to leave by 2:30. My brother Skip was driving me in; my Mother, sister, brother-in-law, and Ann would be coming later. I packed some underwear for at least a few days, not knowing how long I would be in the hospital. My brother Skip picked me up at 2:00, and we headed in. I told him I wasn't frightened, but if anything were to happen to me, I asked him to please take good care of Mom. He dropped me off at the front door and parked the car. I said, "I will meet you in the office adjacent to the operating room."

I walked to the waiting room, and my brother Skip soon joined me there. We were a little early, so we sat down and waited for about thirty minutes. The nurse then came in, introduced herself, and asked Skip and me to follow her to the office. Once there, I answered a few questions and as usual filled out more paperwork. She asked me my name, date of birth, and if I was allergic to anything. She took my vital signs, and we went over my medications. She asked if I had any questions. I said I would like to speak to the anesthesiologist before I was sedated; she said he would be in soon. I thanked her. I was directed into a room to undress and put on a johnny. When I came out, she told me I wouldn't be able to wear my Crucifix and chain for the surgery. I explained to her that it had been given to me by my grandmother in 1960 and, other than the MRIs, I had never taken it off. I asked if she could please check with Dr. Black to find out if I would be allowed to wear it. I also brought a set of rosary beads that I had hoped to hold in the palm of my hand during the operation.

"They won't interfere with anything near my head," I said. "Are they allowed?"

"That won't be a problem, but I will have to check with Dr. Black about the crucifix."

I thanked her.

It was now 3:00 p.m., and I was being prepped for surgery. Another nurse entered the room with a wheelchair, in which I sat. Since Brigham and Women's is a teaching hospital, there was an accompanying nurse who I assume was being trained on how to insert an intravenous needle. Unfortunately, she tried unsuccessfully a few times. At that point, my sister asked her to please stop and let the experienced nurse insert the intravenous needle in my arm and hook me up to the drip. She successfully did in the first attempt. The anesthesiologist entered and asked if I had any concerns. I mentioned to him that my Dad had aspirated a number of times and that was the actual cause of his death. He said he would make sure that my airways were always clear, and he would remain there for the entire operation; I thanked him. It was now 3:30 p.m., and my Mother, sister, and brother-in-law, and Ann had arrived. The nurse came in to tell me Dr. Black had given me permission to keep my Crucifix on during the surgery; I was relieved and thankful.

I could tell the anesthesia was starting to take effect because I was starting to feel drowsy. A third nurse brought out the operating table. I gave everyone a kiss and told them not to worry. I was in God's hands, and He had given me the best neurosurgeon in the world. The nurses assisted me onto the table and then rearranged my Crucifix and chain so that they wouldn't interfere with the surgery. Three nurses, the anesthesiologist, and Ann started to walk me down to the operating room.

I told the doctor and nurses that Ann was a very good friend and my health-care agent. Halfway down the hall, the nurse told Ann that she couldn't go any further and would have to return to the waiting room.

I said, "*Wait! Before you leave*, you know I never call in sick to work even if I don't feel well. Our sick days carry over from one year to the next, so I have a total of three hundred sick days. I plan to be fine, but if I end up on life support, I want you to take out a calendar and count out three hundred school days. As long as I am alive, the checks will continue coming; on day three hundred one, you can pull the plug and wave good-bye."

The nurses and anesthesiologist heard me giggle a little and then started laughing hysterically. I think Ann was too nervous to laugh.

One of the nurses stopped laughing and said, "You haven't had enough anesthesia to not be aware of what's about to take place; do you realize you are going in for major surgery for the removal of a brain tumor?"

"I do."

"Then how can you laugh and tell jokes at a time like this?"

"That's my nature. If I cry, will that help get me through the surgery?"

She replied, "No, not at all."

"Then I will laugh and let God and Dr. Black take care of the rest."

They continued to laugh as I gave Ann a kiss and told her I would see her in a few hours; then they wheeled me into the operating room. I was almost totally under but remember Dr. Black entering the operating room and telling me not to worry because everything would be fine. I am not sure, but I think I heard him ask the nurses what they were laughing about; after that, everything went dark.

THURSDAY, MARCH 25

The operation was over, and I was groggy but alert. I had an IV in my arm and was being monitored for my vitals in what I thought must be the recovery room. A nurse came in and said the operation was complete and that I was in the recovery room and everything appeared to be fine. Then she asked me my name and what I was doing there. I told her my name and said that I had a brain tumor removed; she said, "That's correct."

I asked if my relatives and friends were still here, and she said, "I believe they're still in the waiting room and will be allowed to visit you in a little while."

I thanked her. I said, "My body feels very weak."

She said, "You just had major surgery, and, as Dr. Black explained, it will be weak until you strengthen it with physical therapy."

I felt strange because I was acutely aware of what was taking place. I would have thought that after *major, major* surgery, I would be oblivious to what was happening around me. About fifteen minutes passed, and I asked if I could see my family and friends.

"I will bring them in shortly," the nurse said.

"Thank you."

I was having a difficult time moving, so I asked if she could help me sit up. She called in another nurse to assist her; one held me, and the other propped up the back of the bed. That was the first time I realized I was not only weak but totally paralyzed on my left side and extremely weak on my right side. Never having been through anything like this before, I was unaware of how I was supposed to feel. It was a very strange feeling.

I was anxious to see my family and friends, and after the longest fifteen-minute wait I can remember, they all came in. They were happy, yet amazed, to see how awake and alert I was; they all came over and gave me a kiss.

They asked me how I felt, and I said, "My mind is alert, but my body feels very heavy. I can't move my left side at all, and my right side is very weak, but the nurse said I would gain my strength back through physical therapy." I was totally frightened but did not want to show my fear to my family and friends, especially my Mother.

I thought only six hours had passed since the surgery began, and it must be the middle of the night, but when I asked my sister the time, she told me it was five thirty in the morning.

"Then the operation must have taken a lot longer than they anticipated."

"It sure did," she replied, "and we were here supporting and praying for you the entire time." They asked if I was in pain.

I said, "No, but I imagine I am still on pain medication; I am not sure how I will feel when the meds wear off."

They stayed for another half hour until I said, "All of you have been up for almost twenty-four hours, so please go home; if you want to come back tomorrow, I will see you then. I am doing well and just want to rest." They all gave me a kiss goodbye and reluctantly left.

Looking back, it must have been so difficult for them during the surgery because it took so much longer than expected. Nobody ever came out to explain what was transpiring, so they were extremely mystified about why it took so long. They said they prayed that the procedure was going as planned. As they said to me later, "We assumed no news was good news."

Around 7:30 a.m., I asked the nurse if I could make a phone call; she said, "Absolutely," and handed me the phone. I remembered the number of Kennedy Middle School and made a call. I am not sure who answered, but I said, "Hello, it's Joe Salvo, and I am in recovery."

Whoever answered said, "That's not funny, because last night, Joe had major surgery for the removal of a brain tumor, and this is a bad joke."

I said, "No, it's really me."

"How could you be so alert?"

I said, "My body is hurting, but my mind is sharp."

"Are you sure this is Joe?"

"Of course. The operation lasted about twelve hours, and I am now in the recovery room."

"Wow, Joe, I am shocked. You sound great; it's good to hear from you. I will pass the message on to the rest of the staff that you're doing well."

"Please do, and I will call you in a couple of days to keep you updated."

Now they were ready to roll me up to my room. Two nurses helped me to lie down, and then one grabbed the bed, and the other pushed the IV pole. I made it to my room, which was small but private. The nurse came in and introduced herself.

I said, "Nice to meet you." I asked if I could have a little something to eat.

She said, "Not yet, but you can have a frappe."

Another nurse came in, and we introduced ourselves. Then she washed me and asked me how I felt. I said, "I feel a bit agitated because I am unable to move on my own."

She said, "That will come back with time."

Dr. Black came in to see how I was doing, and I am not sure, but I think it was a reflex hammer that he ran down the bottom of each foot. When he ran it down my right foot, I could feel it a little and told him so. I continued to watch him as he ran it down my left foot and told him I could feel it, even though I didn't; he said, "Fabulous." I was amazed at how alert I was, and as I write this, I am astonished at how much I remember.

CHAPTER 6
THE WORST IS OVER ... OR WAS IT?

As the day went on, I was becoming more and more agitated; my heart was racing, and my insides felt like a volcano ready to explode. I was hooked up to a monitor displaying my blood pressure, heart rate, and pulse. I was lying in one position, and because of the paralysis on my left side and the weakness of my right, I didn't have the power to move or turn. I continually became more unsettled, and by the end of the day, I was ready to jump out of my skin, literally and figuratively. I think it was about 10:00 p.m. when someone turned my light off. After that, I am not sure if it was a dream or real, but I remember sticking my finger and thumb down my throat, trying to pull out my tonsils; I continued this for quite a while. Next, I remember trying to turn over without any luck. I lay there for I am not sure how long and started crying. I was amazed that no one heard me or came in to check on me; if they did, I was unaware of it. It was less than twenty-four hours since my surgery.

FRIDAY, MARCH 26

Why is all of this happening to me? This can't be normal circumstances after removal of a tumor. I have to talk to someone, but no one is around. A few hours had passed, and I had become even more agitated and upset. *What am I going to do?*

As weak as my body was, I remember using all the strength I had on my right side to start throwing anything within reach. I grabbed the cover but could not pull it out of the end of the bed. I held it tight for a couple of seconds and then *threw* it off the end of the bed. I then grabbed the sheet, held it for a couple of seconds, and *threw* that off the end of the bed. Next, I clutched the pillows and with all my strength held them for a couple of seconds and *threw* each separately onto the floor. I then pulled my johnny up but couldn't totally remove it because of the IV drip and monitor wiring. I don't know why I didn't yell or scream for the nurse, but I knew what I was doing was totally irrational. My door was partially open, so I could see the clock from the light that had shone in from the hallway; it was 2:00 a.m., and I hadn't fallen asleep. I was flat on my back now dripping with sweat from exhaustion and fear. I tried to turn over and became terrified because my body was total dead weight. I kept twisting and turning with all my might but appeared to be moving about an inch an hour. I continued to struggle and remember watching the clock, three o'clock, and still not getting any better. Now three thirty and I hadn't moved more than a few inches. *When will this end? I can't live like this any longer.* It was now 4:00, and I was physically and mentally exhausted. *Has anyone been in to see me? Why have I been left alone for such a long time?* Finally, 4:30, and after two and a half hours, I had turned over onto my left side. After all that time, I had finally moved over enough to see the wheelchair that the nurse left directly next to the bed.

I had no idea what was going on and said to myself, *I can't live like this; I have to get out of here* (meaning, this world). I looked at the clock and could see it was almost five. I had used all my strength to pull myself to the left side of the bed, directly beside my wheelchair. I knew with one final pull, I would fall into the wheelchair. I said to myself, *If you don't end up in the wheelchair, you will land on the floor. If that happens, at least you should make enough noise for someone to hear you.*

I grabbed on to the mattress, and with all my strength, I made that *final tug* and dropped into the wheelchair. The IV drip and wires checking my vital signs both disconnected, and I was sitting naked in the wheelchair with my left leg hanging over the side. *Now what do I do? I just want to die.* I noticed the window at the end of the room. The wheelchair had not been locked, so with all the energy I had remaining, I wheeled myself over to the window and tried to open it. The plan was to jump out of the window. I was on the tenth floor of Brigham and Women's Hospital. Fortunately, it wouldn't open, and the nurse finally heard me crying hysterically.[3] She rushed in and said, "What are you trying to do? How did you get out of bed?" She yelled for another nurse and said, "He detached all his wires."

I told her I didn't want to live.

She said, "What's wrong?"

"I don't know. I just want to die."

Still crying, I said, "I have never felt this anxious or agitated before; it feels as if the inside of my body is crawling around trying to get out."

Another nurse came running in, and they lifted me so both legs were in the wheelchair. One wheeled me back to the bed and started putting the bed back together, while the other was reattaching my wires and IV drip. It took a while, but when everything was reconnected, they lifted me up onto the bed, and they both said, "I am not sure what the problem is."

"Before I go crazy, can I please use the phone to call my brother?" I was surprised that they said yes, but I think they would have agreed to anything that would calm me down.

"As soon as we clean you up, you can call your brother." I had been dripping blood from the IV.

---

[3] I had mentioned the experience to family and friends many times without a problem. When I put it in writing, I relived the event, started to hyperventilate, and had to stop writing for a couple of days. Realizing I would have jumped is troublesome.

Once they finished, they handed me the telephone. One of the nurses stayed in the room while I called my brother Skip. I said, "Skip, *please come in and kill me. I can't live like this.*"

He said, "I will be right in," and hung up.

I handed the nurse the phone, and she started to talk, but he wasn't there. She said, "If you continue to act this way, we'll have to strap you in."

I said, "No way," and started yelling. "That will drive me crazy. I will go crazy." It was the worst thing they could have said or done to me because you feel as if you want to be on a raft in the middle of the ocean; being strapped in would have been disastrous.

She said, "We put a call in to Dr. Black; he said he'll be up shortly."

I was still crying when another nurse, Bonnie Manchur, entered the room.

"Why are you crying?" she asked. "And what were you trying to do?"

I explained to her what had happened and said the nurse who just left said she wanted to strap me in.

She said, "Dr. Black should be here soon, and I'll stay here with you until he comes. *You will not be strapped in, I promise you.*"

Shortly after that, Dr. Black entered the room with two nurses. He checked my vitals and said, "He's in a steroid psychosis from the Decadron.[4] He has to be monitored closely for a few days until it passes. He has to be weaned off the Decadron. He has been given sixteen milligrams but shortly will drop to four milligrams. After that, he will have to reduce his intake by a milligram every five days until he has completed the prescription. He'll improve, but he has to take a pill every six hours; if he misses a dose, there's a possibility he could go back into a psychosis." He stayed for a few minutes and then left the room.

---

[4] Decadron, or dexamethasone, is a primary corticosteroid used to control swelling on the brain in patients with brain tumors, defined per a nurse at Brigham and Women's.

The next time I needed Decadron, I would receive four pills of one milligram each, and from that day forward, the dosage would be tapered down one milligram every five days for twenty days. I was feeling very fortunate that Dr. Black wasn't too busy and was available to remedy the situation.

My brother arrived shortly after that. The nurse explained that I was in a steroid psychosis and that Dr. Black was tapering me off the medication causing it. They said I would be closely monitored for the next few days and that it would eventually subside. Skip stayed with me for quite a while, and although I was feeling better, I was still agitated. I told him that it was the worst night of my entire life, and I hoped I never had to go through anything like that again. Bonnie Manchur came back into my room. She said she would keep a close eye on me and reiterated, "No one will strap you in."

At the time, I asked her what her name was in case I needed her. She wrote her name on a little piece of paper, which I still have to this day, and I thanked her.

When you're in a situation like that, it is of immeasurable importance to know that one of the staff is looking out for you. Now that the medical staff realized what I was going through, it was a lot easier for them to deal with me. They were more sympathetic, when, just a short time ago, it seemed as if they were angry enough to open the window to allow me to jump.

As I write this, it's difficult to describe the feeling because it's something I had never felt before. Writing the past few paragraphs was very unsettling because it reminded me of what I had been through.[5]

It was now midmorning, and I was feeling a little jumpy but better. The nurse explained to me what was happening and said Dr. Black informed the staff of the psychosis. As long as I was slowly tapered off the Decadron, I would start to feel better. Although my body was still jittery, mentally and emotionally, I was doing better.

---

[5] I had to stop writing again for two days because it was too emotional.

There was a great sense of relief knowing that, in time, this feeling would pass. I was no longer running on adrenalin, so my body was exhausted. I took a nap for almost two hours and woke up at about 3:00 p.m. At 3:30, my Mom, Patty, and Ann came in to visit; they stayed for about two hours. They heard what had transpired the previous night and this morning and were all very concerned. The nurse explained the psychosis and said I would be monitored twenty-four/seven. That gave them some relief, but they questioned the nurse as to why during my first night postoperation, I wasn't watched more closely; she had no answer. The reason the nurses were unaware of what I was going through was because Dr. Black had his own floor of patients, but that floor was filled, so I was on a different floor. The nurses on this floor apparently had not seen anything like this happen before.

SATURDAY, MARCH 27

The nurse woke me up at 7:00 a.m. to tell me that Dr. Black had scheduled me for another MRI that day. After he read it, he would meet with me to go over the results. I was feeling better, but my lack of control caused me to continue to throw anything in my room within reach. It wasn't looked upon kindly by the nurses, but at least now they understood the reason. I had to repeatedly remind myself that in time, I would be fine, yet nevertheless, I felt very jittery. It was a strange feeling because I was totally paralyzed on my left side and had very little strength on my right side, but the inside of my body felt like a cement mixer.

I started to refocus my energy on exercising, to try to regain the strength and movement that I had lost during surgery. I wanted to get a jump start before I entered rehab. The plan was to use all my time during the day to try lifting my arms and legs; I had slight success on my right side but still no movement on my left. As I mentioned before, I still had enough power with my right arm to throw anything I could get my hands on.

Midmorning a nurse came in to tell me it was time for my MRI. I knew it had to be done, but I was concerned about being in the machine knowing I had to stay perfectly still. I expressed that to the nurse, and she said they thought it would be difficult, so they gave me a pill in my morning medication that would allow me to relax. I said that it must be starting to work because I felt a little less agitated. I made it through the MRI without any problems and then was taken back to my room. A few friends were there when I returned; they said they had arrived about five minutes earlier and the nurse told them I would be back soon. They heard about my frightful night and said they felt terrible for me. I told them thankfully, in time, I would be feeling myself again. During our conversation, I continued working my arms and legs and explained that I wasn't being rude, but this was imperative for my recovery. I still had no mobility on my left side. They totally understood, so we continued our conversation, and they left about an hour later.

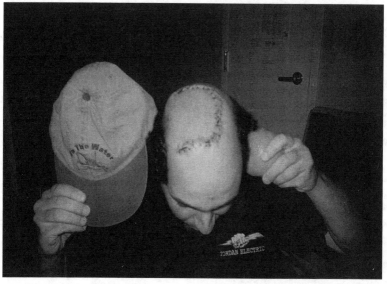

Author perplexed about the size of his tumor - an orange.

Without strength and dexterity, my daily routine activities, such as washing, brushing my teeth, shaving, and eating on my own, were impossible. For the first few days, I was able to use a urinal and a bedpan but would need help from a nurse; it was very humbling and embarrassing.

Early afternoon, Dr. Black entered my room and asked me how I felt.

I said, "Much better than the last two days."

He said, "Even with the three-dimensional MRI, the operation was more complicated and took longer than expected."

I said, "No wonder I woke up in the morning, thinking it must be the middle of the night."

He said, "You made a great decision to have the operation as soon as you did because the tumor was taking up so much space and growing fairly quickly. If you waited even a few more days, it may have snapped the nerve and left you permanently paralyzed. I had to remove it one little section at a time; that's why it took twelve hours. If we pieced it all together, it would have been the size of an orange. I couldn't remove the whole tumor because it was sitting on the nerve, and if I just touched the nerve, it could have snapped and left you paralyzed."

I said, "Great decision."

He said, "I viewed the MRI and read the report, and the results were as expected. I removed the entire tumor except that small piece that was sitting on the nerve. Everything looks clean, but you may still have considerable bleeding."

I said, "Where do we go from here?"

Dr. Black said, "You will soon be transferred to a rehabilitation facility and will receive therapy there until you improve."

I said, "I will work with the therapists as well as work on my own."

He said, "I will set up an appointment for you in a week, and we will discuss the various options."

I said, "Thank you for all you have done."

Dr. Black said, "I will see you in a week," and then left.

Shortly after he left, my Mother, sister, brother-in-law, brothers Skip and Chris, Ann, Father Egan, and other friends and relatives visited. Father Egan led everyone in prayer that I would have a speedy recovery. They all left about an hour later because I was falling asleep.

Saturday night, I slept a little better but revisited what had taken place over the past few days; in hindsight, it felt like a lifetime ago. I knew the members of the medical staff were concerned about me because they frequently checked in on me and left the door to my room open; it was comforting but made it very difficult to sleep.

SUNDAY, MARCH 28

This morning, I woke up tired but said my prayers and was then fed breakfast. The nurse came in to draw blood and give me a sponge bath. I mentioned to her that I was Catholic and asked if there was anyone who could deliver Communion; she said she would check and let me know. She returned twenty minutes later and told me she had contacted a religious layperson and that she would be sending someone to see me soon. In the interim, I started strength training on my own and noticed I could lift my right hand about five inches and left hand about half an inch. It doesn't sound like much, but it was monumental to me. I worked on that for an hour until a nun arrived. We had a short, pleasant conversation, and then she said a prayer, blessed me, and gave me Communion. I thanked her; she said goodbye and left.

When she left, I started to work on my leg-strengthening exercises. My right leg I could move slightly but still no luck with the left. I tried with every ounce of strength I had for at least an hour to just move my left leg but to no avail. It was frustrating not being able to do everything that, before my surgery, was instinctive. I called the nurse in and asked her if I could be transferred to the chair. She called for assistance, and I was moved to the chair. While sitting, I tried to move my right leg forward; I moved it a few inches, but still no movement with the left.

During the day, I had friends and family come to visit. They were all happy to see that the repercussions from my psychosis were subsiding. Prior to coming to my room, they spoke to a nurse who said I would be transferred to a rehabilitation facility on Tuesday. *Thank You, Lord.* I had my best night's sleep on Sunday, especially knowing that I would be leaving in two days.

MONDAY, MARCH 29

I said my prayers, had breakfast, and started contemplating what my future would hold. The following day, I would be going to rehab. I wondered how long I would be there and what the outcome would be; I figured I would know soon enough. My short-term goal was to be completely off the Decadron. I kept track of my medication schedule and knew how many milligrams I was on. Each time I was given Decadron, I would ask the nurse the dosage; I was taking no chances of possibly going back to "la-la land."

During the day, I worked on strengthening my hands, arms, and legs. The in-house doctor came in and said I would be getting a brace to help me stabilize my leg. The nurse came in and measured the length of my left leg. She said she would be back soon. She returned about twenty minutes later with a brace that covered the bottom of my foot and ran all the way to the bottom of my buttocks. It was very restricting, but it kept my leg stiff, which enabled me to stay upright.

I didn't have any visitors until later in the day, so it gave me time to focus on exercising, and I was beginning to see progress. I could lift my right hand about a foot and my left hand only about an inch, but I could tell it was getting stronger. I worked on that for about four hours, had lunch, and then focused on my leg. I had a little more success with my right leg but still no movement from my left; even so, I was still happy with my progress. When I spoke to the staff and visitors, they all commented that they noticed a smile on my face again.

Family members and friends came to visit later in the day, and they all wanted to know how I felt about leaving the hospital; I told them I was ecstatic. I was very appreciative of all the doctors and nurses and what they had done to help me in my recovery, but I wanted to move on and start my rehabilitation. I had dinner around 5:00 p.m., and after dinner, a nurse walked in and asked if I would like a sponge bath to be refreshed for my new home tomorrow. I said that would be great and asked if she could possibly come back in an hour, and she agreed. I spent about thirty more minutes with company, and then they left. The nurse returned about thirty minutes after my company left, gave me a sponge bath, and wished me luck. Knowing I was leaving in the morning, I slept like a log.

TUESDAY, MARCH 30

On the sixth day after my surgery, I was leaving the hospital and heading for parts unknown for who knew how long. I said my prayers and had breakfast, and the nurse came in and took my vitals.

The nurse said, "You will be given a list of medications you will be taking at the rehabilitation facility. Some were inserted in your IV, but now you will be taking them orally or in the form of an inoculation."

I looked at the list and said, "Are you kidding? I don't like taking an aspirin, never mind all these meds."

"As long as you continue to progress, you won't need to take them much longer." I asked if she could list each medication and how they would benefit me.

She said, "Here is the list."

1. Acetaminophen—a common pain reliever / fever reducer.
2. Atenolol—blood pressure medication
3. Decadron (dexamethasone)—a primary corticosteroid used to control swelling on the brain in patients with brain tumors. Has to be tapered down.

4. Colace (docusate sodium)—twice a day stool softener
5. Haldol (haloperidol)—a typical antipsychotic medication
6. Heparin—an anticoagulant (blood thinner) that prevents the formation of blood clots
7. Ativan—used to treat anxiety disorders or anxiety associated with depression
8. Dilantin (250 mg)—taken twice a day, an antiepileptic drug used to control seizures
9. Maalox extra strength—heartburn and upset stomach relief
10. Axid (nizatidine)—used to treat ulcers
11. Simvastatin—used to lower cholesterol

She said the Decadron was the steroid that had resulted in my psychosis. I was being tapered off that and would be totally off it in a little under three weeks. She said the other medications would be stopped as soon as the doctor at the rehabilitation home felt it was appropriate to do so.

I said, "Thanks for explaining everything to me."

She then assisted me in brushing my teeth and shaving. It was around 9:00 a.m. when my Mother and sister walked into my room. We took the elevator down to the first floor at 9:45 a.m. and waited in the lobby for the ambulance. One of the nurses entered the lobby and informed us that the ambulance had arrived. The nurse pushed me out to the ambulance and onto the lift. I thanked her and asked her to please thank the staff. My Mother and sister told me they would follow the ambulance. They had made a note of the name and address of the rehabilitation facility in case they got lost. The ride was uneventful but enjoyable in the sense that I was leaving the hospital and starting on the next phase of my recovery.

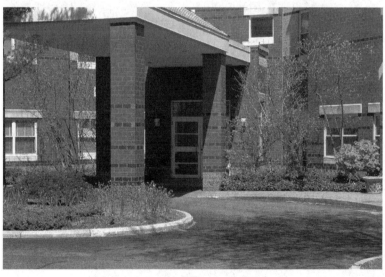

CHAPTER 7
READY FOR REHABILITATION

Main entrance to Wingate at Brighton.

We pulled into the driveway of Wingate at Brighton, 100 North Beacon Street, Allston, Massachusetts, my new home for I was not sure how long. We drove about a hundred yards and then turned right into a small rotary (a roundabout) in back of the building. The driver stopped at the back door of this pretty brick building with well-groomed grounds. The fortunate aspect was that the rehab facility was about twenty minutes from Waltham, where most of my family lived.

The driver stepped out of the ambulance, entered the rehabilitation facility, and two minutes later returned with a staff member, who greeted me and introduced herself. The driver wheeled me out of the ambulance. I thanked him. The staff member took over and wheeled me into the main lobby. It was a large, bright, and colorful room. In the room were a number of chairs and various pictures on the wall. The receptionist / mail clerk was to the immediate left behind the desk. The staff member asked the receptionist to call one of my nurses, and a few minutes later, a nurse entered the lobby.

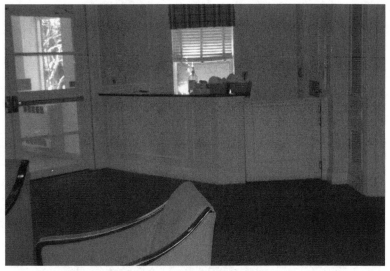

Reception area in Wingate at Brighton.

She introduced herself and said she would be one of my nurses during my stay. I told her my Mother and sister were following the ambulance and would be there soon.

She wheeled me to the elevator, which was around the corner down a small hall. She pushed me onto the elevator and said my room was number 110 on the second floor, which I thought was strange. I was going to say something about 110 being the second floor, but before I could, she said their numbering system was a little bizarre. She said this was actually considered the ground floor, and the room numbers started with a G plus the room number. The second-floor rooms started with a one, and the third-floor rooms started with a two.

We proceeded up to the second floor, took a left out of the elevator, and continued about eighty yards down the hall. Immediately past the head nurses' station on the left was room 110. We entered a bright, spacious room, which was approximately twelve feet by twelve feet with two windows overlooking the back of the building. I could tell it had just been sanitized because of the clean, refreshing smell. Immediately on the left was a chair, and in the far-left corner, there was a built-in nook with shelves and a storage area underneath. The bed was situated in the far right-hand corner about three feet from the back wall with the head of the bed against the wall directly under the light. There was a nightstand with a telephone next to the bed, a bureau in the right-hand corner, and another chair next to the bureau. The door to the bathroom was on my immediate right, and in my opinion, the room appeared very homey. Recently, when I went back to take pictures, I was surprised at how small the room actually was. At the time, I was probably comparing it to the much smaller room I was in at Brigham and Women's Hospital.

Once I was in the room, a nurse arrived. She opened up the curtains and within five minutes gave me a quick sponge bath, washing just my face, arms, and legs. The nurse remained in my room waiting for the rest of the team. Shortly afterward, a team of staff members, including a doctor, nurse practitioner, head nurse, physical and occupational therapist, and social worker entered the room for an evaluation. I assumed they must have had a meeting prior to my arrival because they all came together as a team. Following them were my Mother and sister, who had just arrived; everyone introduced themselves. My Mother and sister sat, and the rest stood.

51

The doctor started the conversation by saying that I would remain on Decadron and be tapered down every five days unless I got bad headaches or neurological symptoms. It was good to hear that they were aware of what had transpired the past week and were just confirming the protocol during my stay. He said other medications would be stopped as soon as he felt they were no longer needed. I never asked what the alternative would be if I did get any side effects from the Decadron. He said blood would be drawn and tested every few days to make sure my organs were not being affected by the medication. The nurse practitioner said I would need 1,200 cc of fluid each day. The head nurse spoke about the rehab staff that would be working with me. She said I would be receiving physical and occupational therapy six days a week for an hour each day starting on Thursday. Each individual therapist would visit me later in the day for an evaluation. A speech therapist would come in to evaluate me, because I was transposing certain words. It wasn't apparent to me, but my sister said that my speech had been slightly altered since my surgery. A doctor and numerous nurses would be onboard for any medical needs. A social worker would schedule all of the team meetings after that day. Then they asked if we had any questions.

I said, *"How soon do you think I will be able to walk?"*

They all looked at each other apprehensively, and before anyone spoke, there was an extended pause of only a few minutes that felt like an hour. This left me feeling very uncomfortable, but they knew I was waiting for some sort of response.

Finally, after what seemed like an eternity, the doctor said because of the size of the tumor and the trauma my body had endured, it would be an uphill battle. The rest of the team remained silent. I said I would work daily with each therapist, as well as on my own, from the time I awoke until I closed my eyes at the end of each day. Strengthening my body and walking would be my primary goals while in the rehabilitation facility; once again, there were no comments or feedback from any team members, which gave me an uneasy feeling.

This entire time I was exercising, trying to raise my left hand and move my left leg. I hoped the team would notice that I was truly committed to my recovery. They said my progress would be evaluated and charted weekly. They left some forms for us to fill out, said their goodbyes, and then excused themselves and left the room. They also gave us a form for the weekly meals, which my Mother filled out, because she said she was aware of my eating habits. She didn't want to upset me but knew that I was still having difficulty focusing and writing. All of this transpired in about thirty minutes, which was quite impressive.

My sister began filling out the forms that were left with us, asking me questions concerning information she was unaware of. To our surprise, the nurse who had remained after the rest of the staff left, knelt down at the foot of my bed, made the sign of the cross, and silently prayed for about two minutes. I was in a state of shock because she really had no idea if I believed in God or not.

I said, "Thank you, but how did you know I was religious?"

She said, "You're wearing a Crucifix, and part of my job is to be observant."

"Thank you," I replied.

She then asked me if I wanted to lie down.

I said, "No, I would prefer to sit in the chair." She called in another nurse, and they transferred me out of the wheelchair and into the chair. She asked if there was anything else I needed, and I said no, that everything was fine. They both said their goodbyes and left. My Mother, my sister, and I all agreed this room was much larger and brighter than my hospital room.

It had only been a few hours since the transfer from Brigham and Women's Hospital to Wingate at Brighton Rehabilitation Facility. It was a relief but totally exhausting; being transported was the most activity I had done since my surgery. Unfortunately, feeling settled didn't change the fact that I was still experiencing anxiety from my steroid psychosis. It was really hard for my Mother and sister to see me this way. I was still being weaned off Decadron. My sister went

53

out into the hall. She mentioned to my nurse that it was time for me to take my pills and asked if she could bring them in. She said she would check and entered my room a minute later with the unsettling news that the order had not been transferred yet. I emphatically said that I needed to take the Decadron, because if I missed a dose, I was at risk of going back into a psychosis.

My sister said, "You have to excuse his abruptness, but if you knew what he had been through, you would understand."

She said she read the hospital report, understood, and would call them and explain the urgency of having my medication transferred as soon as possible. My sister said I was still acting irrationally, which was difficult to see, but I would behave like that until the drug was out of my system. My sister, my Mother, and I were impressed with the staff we had met so far.

The following Sunday was Easter, and my family hoped I would be able to go home for the day, but I asked the nurse before she left, and she said I would have to ask the doctor. I was in the hospital for less than a week and received about fifty get-well cards, so my sister set them up on the bureau and windowsill. My sister and Mother brought in some of my clothes, which they folded and put in the bureau. The room looked cozy and comfortable for a room at a rehab. The nurse gave me a menu and asked what I would like for lunch; I told her just some soup would be fine. She asked my Mother and sister if they would like something, and they declined; they would be leaving soon. About twenty minutes later, lunch arrived, and with the help of my sister, I ate my bowl of soup. Once I finished, my Mother and sister said they were exhausted and would leave as soon as my Decadron was transferred.

My sister said, "I brought in a daily journal for you to keep track of everything that has happened and will take place during your recovery. You will never remember everything unless you write it down." We wrote down what had already transpired in the hospital and from that point on would write down explicit notes on my daily life in the rehabilitation facility.

They didn't say anything, but I could tell by the expressions on their faces that they were still troubled about the whole ordeal that had taken place this past week and were concerned about my future. They called for the nurse to please transfer me into bed, because once my pills arrived, I would take them and then take a nap. The nurse came in, and, with my sister's help, assisted me into bed. The nurse said the prescription should be coming in soon.

I was still almost totally paralyzed on my left side but had enough movement on my right to be able to maneuver my body to the middle of the bed. At about 2:00 p.m., the nurse walked in with my medication—two hours after it was scheduled to be dispensed. I asked my sister to please call Dr. Black's office to explain the delay in taking the medication. Dr. Black was emphatic when he spoke to me about taking my Decadron in order to prevent me from going back into a psychosis. I needed my medication, the correct dosage, and on time. She called Dr. Black's office and spoke to Donna DelloIacono about the two-hour delay. She said it would not cause any adverse reaction and just to continue with the rest of the medication as prescribed. I was still irate about how long it took to transfer the paperwork; I had already been there for five hours. At least now my Mother and sister could leave knowing I was in good hands. They gave me a kiss goodbye and I thanked them for everything. Before they left, I asked them to please send a fruit basket to the staff at Brigham and Women's Hospital in appreciation for the care I had received during my stay.

As tired as I was, I wasn't able to fall asleep. I continued working both arms and legs. I was consistently gaining some strength on my right side but very little progress on my left. There were so many unresolved questions, with no clear-cut answers. To this point, no one offered an opinion as to how long it would take me to walk again. Would I ever be able to walk again? Would I teach or coach again? I had been a baseball and softball coach for a number of years. I finally said to myself, *What are you thinking, you stubborn Italian? Of course you'll walk, teach, and coach again. All it will take is hard work and perseverance, and no one ever died from that.*

The phone rang, and I answered it. To my delight, it was one of my best friends, Gary Rotella, who was a lawyer and owned his own law firm. He was calling from Fort Lauderdale, Florida. He had sent flowers after my surgery, but we hadn't spoken yet. He said he had called the hospital several times but wasn't able to reach me, so he called my Mother. My Mother told me yesterday he had called, and she had updated him about all that had transpired since my surgery, including my psychosis and transfer to rehab. We spoke for a few minutes before he said he had made arrangements to have a friend fly him up to Logan Airport in Boston on Saturday. The plan was to pick me up and take me into Boston for the day. Even though he had spoken to my Mother a few days before, it was obvious that he was not aware of the depth of my immobility. I explained to him that I was paralyzed on my left side and was only able to get around with a wheelchair. He said he would do whatever was necessary to take me into Boston. I thanked him but continued to "state my case" for another fifteen minutes before he realized it would be impossible at this time. He finally relented and agreed to "postpone" our trip to a later date. Gary was a very successful lawyer and was not used to losing an argument. That was the first, and only time, I won a "head-to-head" case between us. We finished our conversation and said our goodbyes, and he promised to keep in touch.

At 2:00 p.m., the physical therapist came in to review some of the questions we had discussed in our initial meeting. She performed a few neurological tests with my arms and legs to check my mobility and strength. These were the same tests my primary-care doctor had originally performed to determine if I needed an MRI. After thirty minutes, she finished up and said she would see me the next day.

About ten minutes later, the occupational therapist followed. At that point, I knew the role the physical therapist would play in my recovery. I was honestly unaware of exactly what an occupational therapist did, but I knew I would find out in the next few days. She asked questions about my living situation: what floor I lived on, if my bedroom was on that floor, and if there was a bathroom on the same floor as my bedroom. I lived in a second-floor apartment in my Mother's home with a kitchen, living room, and bathroom, but my bedroom was on the third floor. She asked a few other questions, but I was exhausted and only half-listening and at the time couldn't figure out why these questions were relevant.

Around three thirty, I needed to use the bathroom and thankfully didn't have to use the bedpan. I did need help transferring from the bed to the wheelchair to the toilet. Two nurses transferred me out of the bed and into the wheelchair and then out of the wheelchair and onto the toilet. It felt good to be sitting on a toilet, as opposed to lying down trying to use a bedpan. When I was ready, the nurses helped me get back into bed. I fell asleep, and at 5:00 p.m., the nurse brought me in another round of pills and said dinner would be delivered shortly. I thanked her and before I knew it, I had fallen back to sleep. I slept for what felt like five minutes. A member of the kitchen staff had delivered dinner. I said I would prefer to eat while sitting in the chair, so she called in a nurse, and they transferred me to the chair. The nurse asked if I would need help to eat; I declined, saying that I could handle it myself. At this point, I was still weak but wanted to try doing more things on my own. It took me a while, and I am not sure what I ate for dinner, but I finished everything on my plate because I was so hungry.

I had just finished my dinner when Skip and Ann arrived for a visit. They both said they were impressed with the room and heard from Patty that the staff was very attentive, and it appeared that things were going in the right direction. Shortly after that, a half-dozen relatives and a friend arrived sporadically to visit and scope out my new temporary home. It was about 8:00 p.m. when I thanked the last two visitors for coming but asked if they would mind leaving so I could get a good night's sleep. The hard work would begin the following day with the goal of regaining the skills I had lost from my surgery.

I needed my life back.

Once they left, I called my sister to tell her I was feeling much better and thanked her again for all she had done. Unfortunately, I couldn't sleep because the constant chatter about my future played over and over again in my head; I was working on trying to get better at turning it off. Even though it had only been a week, with the slight improvement that had occurred, I was hopeful that I would continue to progress.

WEDNESDAY, MARCH 31

The intravenous line had been removed, so any medications would have to be administered in pill form or by inoculation. It felt like I had just fallen asleep when a nurse entered my room and turned on the light that was directly above my head. I think it must have been about five hundred watts, and it startled me.

I said, "This light is bright enough to land a 747 plane; what time is it, and what are you doing here?"

She laughed and said, "I have to give you a shot. You have to receive a shot twice a day, one at 1:00 a.m. and one around noontime."

"For what?"

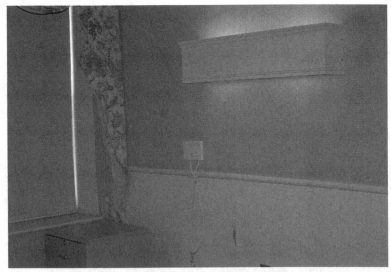

Intense bright light in room 110 in Wingate at Brighton.

"They are given to prevent blood clots. The medicine is called Heparin."

"So, I have to get this shot every night?"

"Yes," she said. "Every night at 1:00 a.m." She came over to my bed and asked me to pull my undershirt up. I pulled up my undershirt. She pinched some skin on my stomach, gave me the shot, and then left. It took about two hours before I could fall back to sleep.

Again, it seemed as if I had just fallen asleep when the nurse came in to give me my meds and tell me it was almost time for breakfast. I said, "What time is it?"

"Seven o'clock."

"It seems like I just fell asleep."

"Well, wake up because you have a big day ahead of you."

Now that I was not hooked up to a machine to display my vitals, I would have my blood pressure, pulse, and temperature monitored each morning during my stay. My aide helped transfer me to a chair, and a couple of minutes later, a kitchen staff member delivered breakfast. That was the first time I had moved from my bed to the chair with the assistance of only one person. After breakfast, I was transferred to the wheelchair and with help brushed my teeth, shaved, and was given a sponge bath. It was around 8:00 a.m. when the aide came in to remove my tray. Once she left, I started feeling anxious again.

My right hand was starting to gain more strength, and I am not sure why, but I reached up to the window shelf, grabbed the get-well cards individually, and *threw* them all over the room. Then I turned around and grabbed the cards off the bureau and *threw* them as well. Then I grabbed the pillows, sheets, and anything else within reach, including the phone, and *threw* them. The phone did make a loud thump when it hit the floor. I then grabbed the clipboard with sheets of my medical information and shredded all the paper onto my sheetless bed. Unlike what happened at the hospital, I kept my johnny on. Even while doing this, I asked myself, "What are you doing?" It wasn't as bad as my first night in the hospital, but all I remember is that I was in an altered state that made me feel as if I wanted to jump out of my skin. Luckily, I couldn't get out of bed and could only throw any object within reach.

My sister came in shortly after and said, "*What did you do?* You trashed the room! Look what you did to your bed, and all these cards I set up yesterday are everywhere." She noticed I was very anxious. I was worried that the two hours that had elapsed yesterday before I took the Decadron was causing me to relapse into a psychosis.

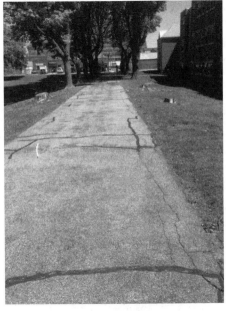

Grounds outside Wingate at Brighton.

I said, "I know it was only a couple of hours yesterday, but that shouldn't have happened. It shouldn't take that long to transfer a prescription."

She agreed but reminded me that Nurse Donna DelloIacono said it wouldn't affect my recovery.

My sister picked up all the cards and placed them on the bureau and windowsill—again. As she was doing that, I began to exercise my left hand. It was the first time she had witnessed this, and she was very excited about my progress. I was now able to lift it about two inches high, which was a great improvement since my initial motion. She brought in lunch for herself and when mine was delivered said, "It's a beautiful day. Would you like to eat outside?"

I said, "Absolutely, if they'll let me."

She asked the nurse if it was okay.

She said, "No problem, just be careful. I will help put him in the wheelchair."

The nurse helped me into the wheelchair, and my sister wheeled me out. It was a beautiful, sunny spring day, so after lunch, she pushed me around the grounds. It was great being outside with the sun beaming down on my face. I noticed the flowers starting to appear. It was a nice feeling to finally get outside for more than the five-minute transfer to and from the ambulance. I asked my sister if she had ordered the fruit basket for the hospital, and she said she did; I thanked her. We stayed outside for another half hour, and then we went back to my room. She stayed for a few more minutes and then left. I knew that I wouldn't be returning to school anytime soon, so I called the substitute service to tell them I would be out for an extended period of time. While I was on the phone, the nurse came in, and as I was talking, she administered my afternoon shot.

The occupational and speech therapists dropped in to see me. At that point, my speech appeared to be fine. When I was having a conversation, it was apparent that I was being understood; no one ever asked me what I had said. I asked the speech therapist why I needed her service, and she said, "You are mildly transposing certain words."

"Whatever," I responded.

I said to the occupational therapist, "It's not an emergency, but could you please contact the doctor and ask him if I could speak to him when he has a free moment?"

She said she would put a call in to him. The occupational and speech therapists each spoke to me for about a half hour; I thanked them, and they left.

The doctor arrived around 2:00 p.m., and I asked him if I would be able to go home for Easter.

He said, "Certainly, just fill out the release form, and whoever picks you up must sign you out and sign you back in."

"Thank you. I know it's only been a week since my surgery, and I feel as if I am making progress, but what is your professional opinion about how long it will take me to walk again?"

"I don't want to be negative"—that was the common response from everyone—"but with a case as severe as yours, you should probably be able to walk with just a walker or cane when you are about sixty years old."

I very loudly said, "*What?*"

He said, "I am only going on past experience with patients in your condition."

I was forty-seven years old at the time and thought to myself, *in another thirteen years, I will be walking with a walker or cane.*

I said, "I hate to disagree, but I will walk out of this rehabilitation facility."

"I wish you were right, but it's never been done by anyone who has had as serious an operation as yours."

"Just wait and see."

He wished me luck and then left.

I called my Mother with the news that I would be home for Easter but never mentioned the doctor's comments about walking.

She said, "Fabulous, I will tell your brothers and sister, and we will have dinner here."

Skip and Ann came walking in around six o'clock and knew I would be home for Easter.

"It will be nice to have you home," they said.

"It will be great to be home," I agreed.

They thought I looked better and noticed I was feeling better. They spoke to Patty and couldn't believe that I had trashed the room that morning. They stayed for an hour and left. During the day, I received a number of phone calls from friends and relatives. I welcomed them but was getting a headache from talking so much. I watched a little television and fell asleep fairly quickly, around 9:00 p.m.

THURSDAY, APRIL 1

I was awakened, yet again, by the nurse at 1:00 a.m. She turned on the light for the arrival of the 747. She administered a shot and left. I woke up around 6:00 a.m. and received a wake-up call from the nurse at 7:00 a.m. I was excited to start working with the physical and occupational therapists and very anxious to see what was in store for me. I had my vitals taken, ate breakfast, and brushed my teeth on my own but needed assistance from the nurse to shave and use the toilet. The nurse asked if I would like a shower.

I said, "I would love one, but I am not sure I could stand."

"You start by taking a sit-down shower with a wheelchair specifically made for that purpose," she replied. "Then I will help you stand to wash your backside."

I have always been very modest, so this was a very humbling experience. She transferred me to the shower wheelchair, set the water temperature, and then gave me my first postoperative shower. It felt great, a little embarrassing, but great. I finished my shower, dried myself, and with the nurse's help, got dressed. I felt like a new person.

The occupational therapist came in at 9:00 a.m. as scheduled. I asked her what role she would play in my rehab.

She said, "I will show you how someone in your condition can have a more fulfilling life."

I wasn't quite sure what that meant; I would have to wait and see.

She said we would have to head down to the first floor, so we took the elevator down to the basement and entered a room that was set up like a kitchen.

She said she read the reports from the hospital and was amazed at how well I was getting along.

"With a tumor the size of yours," she said, "it usually takes weeks before anyone can move at all."

I told her I had the best surgeon in the world, Dr. Black, who did a fabulous job.

"You must be right," she agreed. "Okay, this is what I would like you to do," she began. "With your right hand, unlock the brakes on the wheelchair."

Even that chore was difficult because I had to use my right arm to unlock both brakes. My right hand and arm were gaining more movement and strength each day.

"Now wheel yourself over to the refrigerator with enough room to open the door and then lock your brakes. Now open the door, take out the orange juice, place it on the counter, and then close the refrigerator door. Now we need a glass out of the cabinet. In your house, do you have cabinets below your countertops?"

"Yes, I do."

"Great! Now unlock the wheelchair and wheel yourself to the cabinet. Now lock your wheelchair, open the cabinet door, and grab a glass. Now unlock your wheelchair, and bring the glass over to the countertop where the orange juice is. This is the difficult part because currently you only have the use of one arm."

Getting frustrated, I very loudly asked, "**Why are you showing me this?**"

"If you want to live by yourself, these are the things you will have to learn. If you want any quality of life, for possibly the rest of your life, this is how you will live."

I said very loudly, "***You are nuts.***"

"Joe, this is my profession, and I have never witnessed a patient in your condition walk out of this rehab facility. Some have never walked again without the use of a walker, cane, or brace."

I said, "You obviously have never had a patient as stubborn or strong-willed as I am." I continued to vent, "**No way, I will walk a glass of orange juice down to you and place it on your desk before I leave this rehabilitation facility.**"

"I wish it were true, and not to be mean, but it has never happened."

I played along for the rest of the time, knowing this was nothing I would ever need.

She wheeled me back to my room a little after 10:00 a.m. I thanked her and told her I would see her the next day. I have always been taught to be polite, so I didn't mention anything more about our session.

The physical therapist arrived at 11:00 a.m. and asked me how my occupational therapy went. I said it went fine, but I didn't think it would be much help. Hopefully, tomorrow it would be a little more challenging.

They must have spoken to each other, because she said, "The occupational therapist has to start from step zero and work up from there."

I didn't want to argue and said, "What do you have planned?"

"I would like to have you try to start to take mini-steps."

"That would be great," I replied.

We took the elevator down to a room on the first floor, which had parallel bars along with other gymnastic equipment. She had me wheel myself over to the parallel bars and said, "Now lock your wheelchair. I am going to hold you and have you try to move along on the bars."

"So, you don't want me to flip around like they do in the Olympics?"

She laughed and said, "No, not just yet."

I was at the end of the bars and locked my wheelchair. She helped me up and said, "I will hold you. Just try to at least move your right leg."

I grabbed the right bar with my right hand and draped my left armpit over the bar to my left. Then with total focus, I took a step with my right leg. *What—only four inches?* I was in a state of shock. I tried to move my left leg but had no response, and for the first time, *I was really scared.* I knew that my right leg was very weak, and my left leg was paralyzed, but I visualized my right leg taking a full step and getting slight movement out of my left leg. I am not sure why I had that notion, but I very quickly dismissed it. At this point, I had a few tears run down my cheek, and the therapist asked if I was all right. I told her I would be fine.

When it's something you've done unconsciously since the age of one, it's very disturbing "not to be able to do it."

I had to drag my left leg up to my right by draping my left armpit over the bar, grabbing my left leg with my right arm, and using all my strength to maneuver it forward. I took another small step with my right leg and then repeated the process with my left. I was trying to rush the process, but she said, "Take your time."

I said, "As you know, this is first time I have tried walking, and this is very depressing. I have to start working harder."

She said it was actually better than most, since it had only been a week since the surgery.

We repeated that exercise on the parallel bars three times back and forth with her helping me turn around at the end of the bars. After that, she had me rest for about ten minutes. Then she helped me grab on to a walker and asked me to walk. I walked about six feet, and the results were the same, except that I was able to hold myself up, which astonished me since my left side was still very weak. My right side did 90 percent of the work, and I more or less leaned on the walker rather than hold myself up. Obviously, that was the first time using a walker since my surgery. It doesn't seem like much, but although it was frightening, just taking a few small steps was monumental. I repeated the task a few more times, and then she wheeled me back to my room.

I was still in shock that my right leg, which was my strong leg, would only move four inches. But I was not surprised that I had to drag my left leg up to my right. For as long as I can remember, since childhood, I was always one of the fastest runners with the most endurance. It was disheartening to have such limited mobility. This was my first time trying to walk since my surgery, so to take a step that I thought would be a foot end up being only four inches was difficult to accept. When going through this drill, your brain actually thinks you will be taking a normal stride, but your body won't allow it to happen. At this point, even I questioned whether or not I would ever walk again.[6]

There were about forty more cards delivered to my room from the front desk. I opened and read each one after lunch. While I was reading my cards, the nurse came in and administered my shot. From that day on, except on Sundays, daily I would receive a number of get-well cards.

The social worker came in midafternoon and talked to me for a little while. She said she was going to schedule a team meeting for the next week to check my progress.

I felt better, so all afternoon I sat in a chair and tried to move my left leg. I started by pushing it forward with my right hand, and then moving it independently. I was amazed that it was actually starting to move. Let's not go crazy though; I am talking about only a half inch each time, but it was better than nothing.

My Mother, sister, niece, and Ann came in for dinner around 4:00 p.m. It was Holy Thursday, and they thought that we should eat together. We ordered Chinese food, took the elevator up to the third floor, and ate in the conference room. I said grace and mentioned that without family and friends this would be a very difficult undertaking. My sister added her thanks to the good Lord for my improved health and recovery. My aunt and uncle came in for a visit around 6:00 p.m., and after about an hour, they left. I was exhausted, so the nurse helped me into bed around 8:00 p.m. I fell asleep in the midst of exercising my legs and arms.

I called my brother Skip and mentioned the session that I had with the occupational therapist and how she felt, from her past experience, that I would not walk out of the rehab. I asked him to please not mention this to anyone in the family because it would be too upsetting. He said the staff at the rehab facility were very good, but they should never tell a patient that. I replied that the therapist said it had never been done, and I told her I would be the first.

---

[6] I had to stop writing in the book for the day because I contemplated what my life would be like if I had never regained the ability to walk again.

I was frustrated that I still could not move my toes. I placed my left leg on top of the covers and started talking to my toes, asking them to move. I thought the power of positive thinking might work … *not yet.* I fell asleep shortly after.

FRIDAY, APRIL 2

At 1:00 a.m., I was awakened by the nurse for my shot. I fell back to sleep fairly quickly and then woke up around 6:00 a.m. and waited for breakfast. It was Good Friday, and I had an appointment with Dr. Black that afternoon. My sister and Ann were coming with me to the hospital.

That morning, I had my vitals taken, and after breakfast, I showered and shaved with the help of a nurse but brushed my teeth on my own. I had occupational therapy at 9:00 a.m. and did the same as the previous day: I learned how to pour orange juice into a glass. She also showed me how to dress and undress, with my restrictions. I was very patient but still thinking, *She's nuts.*

I had physical therapy at 11:00 a.m. and worked with the parallel bars and walker. Much to my, and the therapist's surprise, I was actually able to move my left leg about two inches. This was the longest stride I had taken postsurgery. My right leg was also moving at a longer stride, about six inches. The physical therapist and I were both ecstatic with my progress, and I expressed to her that I was working on my own every waking minute. I told her when I first started raising my left hand, I could only lift it about a half inch, and now I could raise it about four inches; now that was progress. As you know, my left leg wouldn't move at all, but now I could move it two inches—more progress.

She said I could walk with a walker as long as there was someone to assist if I needed help. I still had to ask for help when getting in and out of bed. Using a walker was a significant achievement because it would be much easier for me to transfer from a walker to the toilet, as opposed to getting in and out of the wheelchair.

"I am putting in a request for a smaller brace," she said, "because the one you are currently wearing is too cumbersome and restricting your movement. The new brace will only come up to below your knee, which will allow you to have greater maneuverability."

I told her I agreed and asked when it would be available.

She said, "You should have it by Monday."

I thanked her. We took the elevator back to my room. She said goodbye, and I wished her a great weekend. Back in the room, I noticed a number of cards had been left on my bureau. I opened and read them, and two minutes later, lunch was delivered. I ate very quickly, because after all that exercise, I was quite hungry. The nurse arrived and administered my shot in the belly.

A few minutes passed, and a friend called. She said a friend of hers, whom I didn't know, recently found out that she had a brain tumor and needed surgery. She told me her friend went to see the surgeon, and he gave her such a scare that she was a wreck. She wanted to know if I could possibly call her and try to calm her down. I told her I had an appointment with my surgeon that afternoon, but I would give her a call when I returned. She said she would appreciate that very much.

My sister and Ann showed up around 12:45 to take me to my appointment with Dr. Black. I was very excited to tell them about my progress in physical therapy, and they were thrilled to hear the good news. My sister said since I was progressing so well, she had sent in an application for the Boston Marathon on my behalf. I said, "Not this year but maybe in the years to come."

We headed down to the front door, and the ambulance arrived at 1:00 for our 2:00 p.m. appointment at Brigham and Women's Hospital. The driver was very nice, but when he put me in the ambulance, he locked my wheelchair but never strapped the wheelchair to the van. The belts were hanging on the side of the wheelchair, but I figured he knew what he was doing, so I never questioned him. There were seats for my sister and Ann to join me.

We were traveling comfortably at about thirty-five miles per hour when suddenly someone cut out in front of the ambulance. The driver jammed on his brakes to make an immediate stop. I fell forward against the back of the front seat but thankfully braced myself with my right arm, or the wheelchair would have fallen on top of me. Luckily, I was strapped to the wheelchair, or I may have ended up splitting my head open—again. The driver pulled over to make sure I was okay. He apologized numerous times and strapped the wheelchair to the van, which he should have originally done. I said, "My life was saved by Dr. Black, but you're going to kill me. You may be hearing from my lawyer." He was not sure if I was serious or not, so to relieve the tension, I giggled. We all laughed and continued on.

We made it to Brigham and Women's around 1:45. The driver wheeled me out of the ambulance, and then Ann grabbed the wheelchair. We headed up the elevator and sat in the office. We were called in at 2:30 to see Dr. Black, who was accompanied by two other doctors. We all introduced ourselves, and then Dr. Black checked my incision and said it was healing well. He said the tumor was atypical.[7]

He said, "As I mentioned to you last week, if you did not have the operation as soon as you did, it may have snapped the nerve and left you permanently paralyzed. I had to remove the tumor one little section at a time. That's why it was such a long and arduous operation. Do you remember my telling you I could not remove the whole tumor because it was sitting on the nerve and if I just touched the nerve, it could have snapped and left you paralyzed?"

---

[7] Dr. Black states that "atypical" is an official category of meningioma tumors, not just a description (Edward O. Uthman, MD, *This CancerGuide Page*, *patientresource.com*). Atypical meningiomas represent approximately 7 to 8 percent of meningiomas and exhibit increased tissue and cell abnormalities. These tumors exhibit a faster growth rate than benign meningiomas and, on occasion, some degree of brain invasion. Atypical meningiomas have a higher likelihood of recurrence than benign (Brain Science Foundation, Inc.).

I said, "I do, and thank you for making that decision. What course of action do you recommend?"

He said they extracted the tumor but didn't touch any part of the brain because the tumor was encapsulated. During the operation, there was considerable bleeding, so it would be normal if for a while I felt pressure, was dizzy, or was unable to focus.

He added, "Don't get your head wet until your next appointment with me, and in three weeks, you will need another MRI. As it stands now, there is a 50 percent chance for regrowth. To decrease the chance of the tumor returning, I recommend six weeks of radiation five times a week. Radiation will not guarantee another tumor won't grow, but I believe it will decrease your chances of regrowth to only 20 percent."

"I will do whatever you say. Do you have a doctor you recommend?"

"Yes, Jay Loeffler, whom you just met."

Dr. Loeffler said, "It's great to meet you. I work out of Mass General."

I said, "Nice to meet you as well. I assumed I may need radiation so I previously asked Ann, who worked at Waltham Hospital, if radiation was performed there; she said that most definitely it was. Would that be an option, as I am five minutes from the hospital?"

He said, "That would not be a problem. The radiologist there studied under me."

I said, "Great, that will save me a lot of time."

I thanked Dr. Black and then asked him, "How will I know that my brain function is back on track to normal?"

He said, "Once you can *wiggle your toes*, it means the brain has sent a signal to the furthest part of your body, and you will be on your way to strengthening your left side."

After thanking him, we all said our goodbyes and left around 3:30 p.m.

I was becoming agitated because it was time for me to take my Decadron. The medication could only be dispensed at the rehab facility, so we didn't have it with us. We called for the ambulance, and in the meantime, I asked my sister to wheel me around the hall because I needed to be in constant motion. The movement stimulated my body, so she pushed me up and down the hall until the ambulance arrived at 4:15. Because of the time lapse in receiving my medication, I feared going back into a psychosis. The driver said slow traffic was the reason for his delay. We all got into the ambulance and headed back to rehab.

It took over an hour to get back to the rehabilitation facility, and by that time, my body felt like it was ready to jump out of my wheelchair. As we passed the nurses' station, I talked to the nurse about my pill.

She said, "I will bring it to you shortly."

As soon as we arrived back in my room, I said, "I have to take my pill."

In five minutes, the nurse delivered the pill to my room, and in thirty minutes, I felt fine. At that point, my sister and Ann said they were exhausted and had to leave.

I thanked them and said, "Please call Skip and tell him I am tired and prefer not to have company tonight; I am drained." I had dinner and then relaxed for a few minutes.

Shortly after dinner, I called my aunt Lorraine, who was a nurse. Her husband, my uncle Carmen, was my Mother's brother. I told her about Dr. Black's recommendation to have radiation and then mentioned having it performed in Waltham.

She said, "No way. You will go to Boston and only Boston, no matter what it takes. If you can't find a ride, somehow we will get you there."

I said, "But Dr. Loeffler said the radiologist in Waltham had studied under him and that would be acceptable."

She said, "Dr. Loeffler does this all day because of the number of patients who go to Boston hospitals for brain injuries. How many patients have brain surgery in Waltham and then end up staying there for radiation? The radiologist in Waltham is probably a great doctor but would not have the skills of Dr. Loeffler."

She made a lot of sense.

Another comment that helped me finalize my decision to go to Boston came from a friend of mine who was also a nurse. I mentioned to her I had to have radiation and told her my plans were to have Dr. Loeffler treat me.

She said, "You didn't hear it from me because I work for a different radiologist and would be fired for telling you this, but Dr. Loeffler is the best in the world."

So, the decision was made. I would call Dr. Loeffler in the morning to tell him of my decision to go to Boston.

At 6:30, I called the person afflicted with the brain tumor my friend had asked me to call. She was crying when she answered the phone, not even knowing who was calling. I introduced myself and said that I had just had major surgery for the removal of a brain tumor and that I was doing very well. I didn't mention anything about the psychosis because I didn't want to frighten her. I asked her why she was so upset, and she said it was because her surgeon told her she may not make it through surgery.

"What? That's crazy. Why would he say a thing like that? No one should ever say anything like that to you, especially someone in the medical field. What exactly did he say?"

"He said that because it continues to grow, I definitely have to have it removed. He explained that brain surgery is very serious and with that type of operation ..."

She couldn't finish her sentence.

I said, "Okay, take your time and take a deep breath."

She waited about a minute and said, "He told me that it was growing in a bad spot and that I could possibly bleed out on the table and not make it through the operation. He said if I do make it through the operation ..." She once again couldn't finish, so I reminded her to take her time and take some deep breaths.

She continued, "If you do make it through the operation, you will have a difficult time in recovery."

She continued crying, and I said, "That's insanity. This doctor should be reported and not be in the medical field. You have to get another doctor."

She said, "My husband was with me, and I left him and ran out of the office. I was crying hysterically."

"I don't blame you."

"My husband followed shortly after and consoled me."

"How large is your tumor?" I asked.

"About the size of a peanut."

"The size of a peanut. That's a baby. Mine was about the size of an orange, and I am doing fine."

"But mine might be in my brain."

"Did he say that?"

"No, he just said it's in a bad spot."

"After what you just told me, you need to call the hospital first thing tomorrow morning. Explain to them that because he said you definitely need surgery, you would like to request a second opinion. Just stay positive, and have a glass of wine tonight. After you call and meet with the other neurosurgeon, if you still feel uncomfortable, call me back."

She said she felt better talking to me and would call the hospital the next morning. We both said our goodbyes and hung up. After that story, I felt even more fortunate to have had Dr. Black.

I realize doctors have to explain all the possibilities in any procedure, but my opinion is her doctor described the worst-case scenario in order to look good if she came through her surgery without any problems.

I watched television for a little while, talked to my toes, and asked them to move, but they were being stubborn—no such luck. I fell asleep around 8:00 p.m. and slept like a log.

That Friday was a very long day, so my sister wrote the day's quote, attributed to Mignon McLaughlin, in my journal: *The only courage that matters is the kind that gets you from one moment to the next.*

SATURDAY APRIL 3

I was administered my 1:00 a.m. shot and then fell right back to sleep. I woke up around 6:00 and was given breakfast at 7:00; then my vitals were taken. The nurse brought in my pills, and I noticed there was only one Decadron.

I asked why I was receiving only one, and she said, "That's what the prescription calls for."

"No, I am supposed to get two."

She insisted it was only one, but I emphatically stated that wasn't the case; it was two.

After a few minutes of disagreeing on the number of pills I should take, I said, "Please call the head nurse."

A few minutes later, the head nurse came in, and I told her, "The nurse and I disagree on the number of Decadron I am to receive; she says one, but I know it's two. Dr. Black said if the Decadron isn't followed exactly as prescribed, I could go back into a psychosis.[8] Could you please check the hospital referral form?"

The head nurse said, "Certainly," left for a few minutes, and came back with a second pill. She asked the nurse, "How did you come up with one pill?"

She said, "I am not sure; I think I may have subtracted two from three and came up with one."

The head nurse said, "All you had to do was to check the referral form."

In the hospital and rehab facility, I realized that you have to be an advocate for yourself and be aware of what is taking place, because people are human and make mistakes. What she did made no sense at all.

---

[8] Dr. Black stated that as long as I went from four to three to two to one pill my health would steadily improve. Even if I went from three to one, I could return into a psychotic state. Because being in the psychosis was so devastating, I kept strict track of the number of pills I had taken.

"Thankfully, Joe was aware of the situation, or he could have, once again, slipped into a psychotic state. We'll talk about this later in my office."

They both apologized and then left.

I brushed my teeth and for the first time shaved on my own. With the help of a nurse, I showered, transferred to the toilet, and got dressed for physical therapy. Because of my progress, I convinced both therapists to allow me to use both hours for physical therapy instead of occupational therapy for an hour and physical therapy for an hour. The occupational therapist would now be working with me on physical therapy. They were both very pleased with my progress and said it was a miracle. Neither of them had ever seen anyone with such a massive tumor walk as well as I had in such a short period of time. It had only been one and a half weeks since my surgery. I attributed my "miracle" to my strong will and constant exercise.

I began to wonder when and what skills I needed to master in order to go home. Although I was progressing well, I knew it would still be quite a while.

My Mother, sister, niece, and brother-in-law brought in lunch, which we brought outside to eat. I told them about my progress in physical therapy, and my sister asked if I could "wiggle my toes" yet.

"Not yet, but hopefully soon," I replied.

After lunch, they stayed for a little while and then left knowing I would be coming home the next day for Easter.

A staff member came in and dropped off a few more cards. The nurse then came in and administered my shot. In the afternoon, Father Egan came in to visit. He told me a few jokes, which he rattled off one after another. He had no problem remembering jokes, which always amazed me because I would usually forget a joke by the next day. He was such a great person, and as I would tell friends, he was a "priest's priest," meaning he was a priest all the other priests looked up to. He blessed my scar, prayed for a speedy recovery, and then left around 3:00 p.m.

I continued exercising and was standing up using a walker when Ann arrived. She was shocked to see me standing and taking small steps and said, "This is very encouraging."

I said, "Each day, I am getting stronger and walking a little better."

Skip and his son walked in around 5:30. I told them about my progress and made arrangements for him to pick me up the next day; we had a good conversation, and they left around 6:30. A couple of friends came in soon after and stayed for about an hour. I went to bed at 8:00 p.m. and watched television for about a half hour. I was exhausted but couldn't fall right to sleep because I was excited about going home tomorrow for the day.

SUNDAY, APRIL 4

I was administered my 1:00 a.m. shot and then fell back to sleep. I woke up about 5:00 a.m., anxious to go home for Easter. I am not sure if it was the fact that I was able to go home for Easter or I was just improving, but I felt the best I had felt postsurgery. I got out of bed on my own for the first time and took a few steps with the walker. I walked to the chair and sat down. The nurse came in at 7:00 and was furious. "Who helped you out of bed?"

It was Easter, so I had to tell the truth.

"No one," I said.

"Anytime you have to get out of bed, you must let us know, and we'll come in to help. If you ever fell and hurt yourself, I could lose my job."

"I am getting stronger and have to start becoming more independent."

"Until you get permission from the doctor or head nurse, you have to call us. Now take a shower, shave, have breakfast, and get ready to go home for the day."

The head nurse instructed her staff that a nurse would no longer have to accompany me into the bathroom but must be present in my room in case I needed help or fell. I now had the ability to stand on my own in the shower and wash myself while holding on to the safety handles, a situation that was definitely less embarrassing.

The staff would never intentionally impede my ability to advance, but I felt as if I was progressing faster than they thought I could. I finished my morning routine and was anxiously awaiting my ride. Skip showed up at nine. I decided to use my wheelchair, as opposed to the walker, to make the trip home easier. I went to the front desk, where I had to be signed out. The head nurse confronted me about getting out of bed on my own.

"Please don't do that again, and have a good day."

"Thank you, and 'Buona Pasqua.'"

She said, "What does that mean?"

"It means 'Happy Easter' in Italian."

Skip wheeled me out to the car and then lifted me up into a brand-new Toyota 4runner.

I kiddingly said, "Wow, when did you buy this?"

He said, "I am only borrowing it until a certain brother of mine gets permission to drive."

"Just don't forget who it belongs to." It was actually my car that I had purchased just a couple of weeks prior to being diagnosed with my brain tumor. I told Skip he could drive in luxury until I received permission to drive.

We arrived at around ten to a beehive of activity: family, friends, and neighbors. I was so excited about spending the day at home! *Hallelujah*! I received a few bouquets of flowers, as well as a fruit basket, from my extended family and friends who couldn't be there. I spent most of the time telling visitors about the gains I had made over the past few days. They were very excited and pleased to hear about my progress.

Another group of friends and neighbors showed up between eleven and eleven thirty to extend their greetings and left around noon to be with their own families. We wouldn't be eating for a couple of hours, so I had some taganu (pronounced ta-ah´-noo) to hold me over.

Taganu is a traditional and very rich pasta dish, originated by our ancestors for the Easter holiday. When I was young, I always assumed it was an Italian dish, but native Italians to whom I spoke had never heard of it. Then I presumed it may have had its origins in Sicily, but a number of Sicilians had not heard of it. Finally, I asked someone whose ancestors were born in the same town as my Mother's ancestors and discovered they were aware of the tradition. I looked up the original recipe to discover it originated specifically in Aragona, Sicily, from where my Mother's ancestors immigrated. Depending on the size of the pan you are cooking it in, it can contain anywhere from one to two pounds of rigatoni pasta, one to two dozen eggs, and one to two pounds of various cheeses depending on the recipe. The recipe is centuries old; it is a very satisfying meal featuring ingredients that were readily available in those early days. Our ancestors were all farmers, even if they didn't practice agriculture for a living. Some of the richer ancestors would add meat to their recipe. The recipe has changed over the years, but no matter how it was made, it's delicious. Look up the recipe on the internet; taganu of Aragona.

My Mother had nine siblings, and our families all lived within walking distance of each other. Every Easter, each aunt would make taganu. All the cousins conspired to go to each aunt's house and tell her that her taganu was the best. We told each aunt not to mention it to any of the other aunts because they would be upset. Each aunt was always so proud to think they made the *best* taganu.

Shortly after noon, we had our family Easter egg hunt, which I hosted each year. I supplied the funds and candy for the eggs and usually hid them on my own, but this year, I needed help from my brothers and sister. My nieces and nephews had a great time competing to find the most eggs. After the Easter egg hunt, my cousin gave me a much-needed haircut; then it was time to "mangia" (Italian for "eat").

Joseph C. Salvo

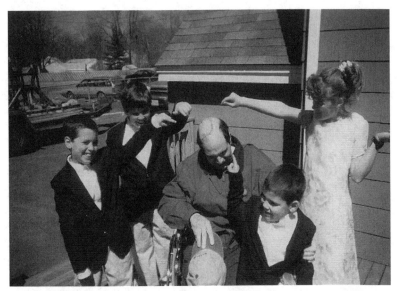

Author being the center of attention with his
niece and nephews on Easter Day.

I said grace, thanking God for placing me in the care of such wonderful family and friends, who had been there for me unconditionally. Each person contributed in his or her own way to help me through the surgery and now the recovery. It was a very emotional moment.

Now for the food. We started with ravioli, which is my favorite, then ham, sweet potatoes, vegetables, and ricotta pie for dessert.

In the afternoon, Father Egan visited to bring me Communion; I was very appreciative. We spent a few minutes talking about how my faith had helped see me through this experience with hope and no fear. He stayed for a little while longer and then left. The day couldn't have been any more beautiful.

After a day of blessings, my brother Skip drove me back to Wingate at Brighton. I was physically and emotionally exhausted. After checking in at the front desk, I dropped off some taganu for the nurses. I explained the tradition and said, "Please try some, and I know you will enjoy it."

80

I was resting in bed by seven thirty, reflecting upon what a blessed and joyous Buona Pasqua it was, being surrounded by such loving family and friends. I fell asleep around nine.

MONDAY, APRIL 5

I was awakened by my nurse at 1:00 a.m. and administered my shot, and I fell right back to sleep and slept until 7:00 a.m. when the nurse entered my room. I really didn't do anything strenuous on Easter, but the experience was nonetheless draining. I started the day with my regular routine and then got ready for physical and occupational therapy. Now that I had started to take small steps with my walker, my therapists began working in tandem to concentrate on my walking skills. I think the occupational therapist realized I was serious when I said I would walk out of there.

The physical therapist said, "Your new brace is in. You can keep the old one for a souvenir, but this new one will be much less cumbersome."

I put it on; it was less restricting and much more comfortable.

I walked with my walker down to the elevator and then to the physical therapy room and worked out on the parallel bars. Afterward, both therapists mentioned my steps had increased to about seven inches with my right leg and four inches with my left. They were thrilled with my progress. They said they had never seen a patient, two weeks post-op, progressing at such a steady rate. I reiterated that every waking moment, I was exercising; they replied that it was still incredible.

I wasn't given the liberty to walk alone with my walker, so when I returned to my room, I asked the nurse if I could go outside in my wheelchair. She told me that was fine as long as I was careful, so she assisted me into the wheelchair (even though I could have done it on my own). I pushed myself onto the sidewalk and around the grounds. I wheeled myself to the front gate, which was locked, and watched as the cars drove by. It was difficult to see because my thoughts were that I should be outside driving one of those cars, not here in a wheelchair. How my life had changed over this short period of time! Then my mind immediately went to that uncertain place, questioning if and when I would drive again.

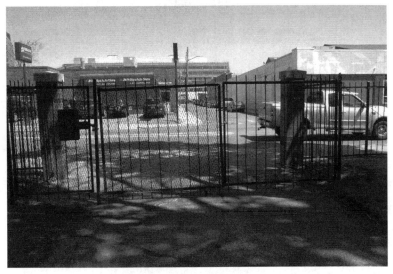

Author staring at traffic on N. Beacon St. in front of
Wingate at Brighton and becoming emotional.

It made me realize how often I take everyday things for granted; one doesn't know what one has until it's lost. I am not sure why, maybe because of the Easter season, but I became very emotional and started to cry while staring out at the traffic. I knew how blessed I was to be alive and have such wonderful, supportive family and friends, but occasionally, I became emotional, and this was one of those moments.

After being outdoors for a few hours, I wheeled myself back to my room. Shortly after I returned, the nurse arrived to administer my shot. Not too long after, the head nurse and a nun visited. The head nurse said the nun had asked her if she knew of anyone who might want Communion on Easter Monday. "I immediately thought of you," the nurse said.

We introduced ourselves. She said a short prayer, blessed me, and then gave me Communion. She then said, "I have to make other visits, so have a blessed day."

She left, but the head nurse remained in my room. She said, "Just to give you advance notice, we have another meeting scheduled for Thursday, April 8."

I thought, *there must be more to this visit than to just inform me about the meeting. Is she going to lecture me for getting out of bed? Why is she still here?*

She said, "Joe, the therapists told me you're taking steps with your walker." She had not seen me because she only worked weekdays, and I went to see Dr. Black on Friday.

I said, "They're small steps but steps nonetheless."

She asked if I would demonstrate it for her. I agreed, so she helped me with my walker. I took a few steps, turned around, and walked back and sat in the chair.

She said, "Do you realize that this is a miracle?"

I said, "I never considered it a miracle because I have been working with such intensity, it never entered my mind. The true miracle is how everything fell into place prior to my surgery, having Dr. Black as a surgeon, and having such wonderful family and friends."

"Joe," she said, "I have been doing this for many years and have never seen anyone in your condition walk out of the rehabilitation facility. Most patients, with the severity of your surgery don't walk for years without a walker or cane. You may be the first to walk out of here, so continue doing whatever you're doing."

"I truly didn't think I had done anything special, but from the attention I am getting from the staff; I guess I did."

"So, do you think your room being right next door to the head nurses' station was just a coincidence? Through no fault of anyone at Brigham and Women's Hospital, because of your surgery and psychosis, they requested your room be right next to the head nurses' station. Seldom do I get that request. We moved a patient out of this room so that it would be available for you. I can't stress how shocked, as well as proud of you, we are, for all you have accomplished. You're an inspiring success story, so continue to work hard."

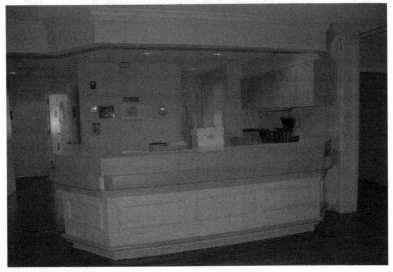

Head nurses' station adjacent to the author's room. Not a coincidence.

"I will."

"Great." Then she left.

In the afternoon, I decided that in order to maintain or accelerate the rate of my progress, I needed to have fewer visitors. I was working out with visitors here but not with the same intensity. I couldn't tell my family and close friends not to visit. I did have some colleagues from school visit and mentioned others were planning to come in. In order not to hurt anyone's feelings, I called the school and told the secretary to relay to the staff that the doctor suggested I cut down on the number of visitors. I felt bad but getting back to walking was my number-one priority at that time.

My room overlooked a softball field, so through the week, I watched pickup softball games being played. That day, I looked out and noticed what I believed to be a school team dressed up in what appeared to be practice uniforms. They may have been playing for

Brighton High School, but I never inquired. I just enjoyed watching them and wondered whether I would ever coach again. Would I ever be able to hit infield practice, and if not, would players ever respect and listen to me? Anytime I questioned myself, I immediately turned it around and said to myself, "Of course, I will; it will just take time." Not knowing the landscape, I found out years later that Mt. Saint Joseph's school was bordering the property of Wingate at Brighton and facing the street parallel to the rehabilitation facility. The team was the Mt. Saint Joseph's girls' softball team.

Ann, Skip, and a friend came in around dinnertime and brought me a pepperoni pizza. I ate a few pieces and then ate a chicken sandwich, which was that night's dinner from the kitchen. They gave me great news that the woman I spoke to a few days ago with a brain tumor found a new surgeon, had the surgery, and was doing very well. I said, "That was quick. I spoke to her just a few days ago." They told me she found a surgeon, had an appointment with him the next day, and was operated on the next morning. It reminded me of my situation with Dr. Black: I had an office visit on a Tuesday and surgery on Wednesday.

We had a lot of laughs during their visit, and after a couple of hours, they left. During the day, I received a half-dozen phone calls and started to contemplate having my phone disconnected. The phone calls were also starting to interfere with the main task at hand—to walk as I did prior to my surgery. I went to bed around 9:00.

TUESDAY, APRIL 6

I was administered my 1:00 a.m. shot and fell back to sleep. I woke up at 6:00, and the nurse came in at 7:00.

She said, "How can you always be in such a good mood?"

"I find it easier to smile and laugh than to frown and cry," I replied.

"You have a great attitude."

"Thank you." I ate my breakfast and then completed my daily morning routine.

I had physical therapy from 8:30 to 10:00 because I had to leave for the hospital by 11:00 to have the stitches on my head removed. The two therapists conferred and decided that, even though I was walking very slowly with my walker, my balance was good enough for me to walk with my walker on my own in the rehab facility. I was ecstatic, because I had been doing it on my own, but now with permission, it was, so to speak, "legal." I asked about getting in and out of bed on my own, and they wanted to see me perform that task a few times before they would make a recommendation to the head nurse. I said, "Let's try it now."

They both agreed. I performed the task with little effort a few times, going from my bed to the walker and from the walker to my bed. They both said they would make the recommendation but to please be very careful. I asked if they could ask now. They said they would, left for one minute, came back, and gave me the much-coveted permission. That was a major breakthrough, because I had been calling a nurse to help me in and out of bed if I needed to use the bathroom, a seemingly insignificant task I had done for forty-seven years.

Ann and my Mother arrived around 10:45. I was grinning from ear to ear. They asked me what was up. I said that I was walking independently with my walker around the rehab and could get out of bed without assistance.

"Wonderful," my Mom said, "but we have to get going. The ambulance will be here in fifteen minutes."

I cleaned myself up and then sat in my wheelchair. We all went down in the elevator, and two minutes later, the ambulance arrived. It was a different driver than the one who transported me to see Dr. Black. I told him about my experience when the driver forgot to buckle in my wheelchair. Unfortunately, he had to jam on his brakes, and the wheelchair partially fell over. He asked if I had filed a complaint.

"No," I said. "He appeared to be such a nice man that I didn't want to get him into trouble."

"You're very kind; hopefully he learned a lesson."

We made it to Brigham and Women's on time. I sat in the waiting room for about ten minutes, and then I went into the office and had the stitches removed; it was a painless procedure. We called for an ambulance to transport us back to Wingate at Brighton. The whole routine took only a few hours. When we returned, Ann and my Mother wheeled me to the elevator and then up to my room. They said they had to leave, so we said our goodbyes, and they left.

The nurse came in and administered my shot. Shortly after, two nurses, one whom I had seen on my floor and the other I didn't recognize, entered my room and asked if I would be willing to answer a few questions.

"Absolutely," I said. So, they questioned me.

At first, they wanted to know how I was feeling and to what I attributed the miraculous gains I had made in just a week's time in rehab. My answer was that I worked on my physical therapy regimen every free moment since my arrival. The interview took about twenty minutes, and they were writing down my answers word for word. Occasionally, they would ask me to repeat my statements. Looking back, I wasn't inquisitive as to the reason for the questions and notetaking. Having never been in a rehabilitation facility, I just assumed it was protocol. I found out years later that this was not the norm for every patient. The phone rang a couple times during our conversations, but I just ignored the calls.

I had a few visitors later that night, including my brother Skip and two friends. I also received a couple of phone calls, one from a cousin that nobody in my family ever heard from. I mentioned that to Skip and his response was "Wow, you must be on your deathbed."

I was glad I notified the school that I wasn't receiving visitors because, between family and a few close friends, my room already had a revolving door. In order to continue to improve, I had to work with as few interruptions as possible.

I hadn't had a bowel movement for the past few days and was experiencing bad stomach pains. I attributed it to all the cheese and ricotta I had consumed on Easter and possibly my medication. I notified the nurse, and she said if there was no movement soon, she would have to give me an enema.

An hour passed and still no defecation. She said that she would have to go through with the plans for an enema. I pleaded for a little more time, but thirty more minutes passed with nothing, so I was given an enema.

Still no luck. She said, "I think you need to go to the hospital."

"Please, just give me a little more time." She did, and fortunately, about thirty minutes later, it happened. *What a relief!*

I said my prayers and fell asleep immediately after, which was amazing considering what I had been through the past few hours.

WEDNESDAY, APRIL 7

I was administered my 1:00 a.m. shot. I was now two weeks out from surgery. Each morning, I continued with my tandem physical and occupational therapy sessions. It was a beautiful day, so my therapists decided that because I was doing so well, we would go outside with my walker. We walked for about an hour, and they showed me how to go up and down the curb or stairs. "If you're stepping down," they said, "you lead with your left foot; if you are stepping up, you lead with your right. To remember that practice, we tell patients, 'You *left* to go down toward hell, but you go *right* up to heaven.'"

I laughed and said, "I think I can remember that. What's the reasoning behind using a different foot when you go up or down?"

"Your right foot is stronger, so when you're stepping down with your left, you want to keep your right foot for stability. When you're stepping up, you need your stronger foot to push off with."

"That makes sense," I said.

My brother Skip showed up, greeted us, and joined us outside. We stayed outside for another half hour; then we went back to my room, and my brother left.

Once we had arrived back in my room, I said to the physical therapist, "Because this is your specialty, I have a question for you. My right leg is continually getting stronger, but I find my left leg is depending upon my right leg to take a step. What exercise would you recommend I add to my routine to help strengthen my left leg?"

She said, "Lie in bed on your stomach, and with your right hand, pull your left leg up to a ninety-degree angle, and then very, very slowly allow it to fall back into a straightened position onto the bed. Continue with that exercise for as long as you can, and all the muscles in your leg will start to strengthen."

"Thank you; I will try it this afternoon and will tell you how well I did tomorrow."

The nurse came in and administered my shot in the belly, and shortly after, I ate my lunch.

I was excited to try out my new exercise when the phone rang. Before I answered it I thought, *This is crazy. I am never going to get better if I have to keep answering this phone.* It was my Mother, who wanted to know how I was doing.

I said, "I am doing well, but I get about twelve calls a day, and it's very disruptive when I am trying to exercise. Please tell family and friends that I appreciate their phone calls, but I am unplugging my phone during the day because it's interfering with my progress. If they want to talk to me, please call after 6:00 p.m."

"How will I get a hold of you if there's an emergency?"

"I doubt there will be any emergencies that I could help you with in my condition, but if there is, just call the head nurse."

She was a little upset because we usually spoke a few times a day, but right then, my priority was to get stronger. Family and friends continued to visit, but predominantly at night, which would allow me to proceed with my strenuous exercise routine during the day.

After we spoke to each other, I unplugged the phone and lay down on the bed on my stomach to start my new exercise. During lunch, I had been watching the noon news and did not turn off the television for my exercise. I pulled my left leg up to a ninety-degree angle and then very slowly allowed it to fall back onto the bed. As soon as it hit the point where the weight of my leg was too heavy, gravity took over, and it just *fell* onto the bed. I was trying to concentrate on having it decline at a very slow rate but each time ended up with the same results. It was very frustrating, but I kept trying. I told myself, "Now focus and put all your thoughts into slowing down." I tried at least a hundred more times with no luck. I am doing exactly what she told me to do, so why am I having such a problem with this exercise? Maybe my leg is still too weak, I thought to myself.

The rest of the afternoon was quiet, especially without any phone calls. Three other nurses who were strangers came in at different times with pen and paper. They were aware that when I arrived at the rehab facility, I was paralyzed on my left side and partially paralyzed on my right. Each questioned me using different terminology but asking basically the same questions.

The most important question was, "How have you progressed to this point in such a small amount of time? What do you do during the day for PT and OT? What do you do on your own? How are you able to walk in such a short period of time?"

I gave them all my standard answer: work. I explained what I meant by work—lifting my arms as far as I could and moving my legs back and forth as much as I could. I said, "When I first started, I was unable to lift my left arm at all. I then progressed to about a half inch, and now I can lift it almost a foot. My right arm has approximately three-fourths of the strength and mobility it had prior to the surgery. After the operation, I could only slightly move my right leg, and now I can take almost a full step. My left leg had no strength, and wouldn't move even a half inch, but now I can step about four inches."

They congratulated me and thanked me for my time. Before leaving, one nurse said, "You really are a 'miracle.'"

Once again, I thought this whole process was unusual, but yet again, I assumed that this was standard protocol for every patient to chart his or her progress. As I look back, I am not sure why I never bothered to ask any of them what the purpose of their visits was.

CHAPTER 8
DID SOMEONE MENTION
MY GOING HOME?

THURSDAY, APRIL 8

I was administered my 1:00 a.m. shot and then woke up at 6:00, anxious to speak to the physical therapist about the issues I was having with my exercise. I went through my regular morning routine, starting at 7:00. When I was done, I jumped (not really) on the bed, lay on my stomach, and tried my new exercise again, still with no luck. That afternoon, the therapists had scheduled a 1:00 p.m. team meeting.

It was 9:00 a.m., and the therapists entered my room and told me I was walking so well with a walker they would like to have me try walking with a four-legged cane. I was delighted and excited, yet a little nervous without showing it. They took my walker, handed me the cane, and asked me to walk the hall. I walked back and forth down the hall as they held on to me. I was a little unsteady, but thought I did a terrific job, considering this was the first time back on my feet with only minimal support. I was told that until I gained enough strength in my legs, I would need someone with me for assistance. They said I could use my cane if there was someone around for support; otherwise, I was to use my walker. I thanked them, and after I walked back to my room using them as an aid, they said they would see me at 1:00 p.m. for the meeting.

I said to the physical therapist, "Before you leave, I have to tell you that I was unsuccessful with the exercise you gave me to strengthen my leg." I explained the procedure and told her I must have tried it at least 150 times, and gravity took over every time my leg hit about a 45-degree angle; it was very frustrating.

She asked, "Were you totally focused?"

I said, "Totally."

She said, "Were the shades up?"

"Yes."

"Was the television or radio on?"

"Yes, the television."

"Were the lights on?"

"Yes."

She said, "Then you weren't totally focused."

"But I'm telling you I was."

She explained, "This is what I want you to do: close the door, turn the lights off, turn the television and radio off, pull the shades down, and then try your exercise and let me know the outcome."

"I will give that a try after the meeting and let you know the results tomorrow," I replied.

As soon as she left, a nurse came in to draw some blood. This was done a few times each week to make sure the medications weren't affecting my organs. After, I worked out, washed, ate lunch, and was eager for my meeting. The nurse came in shortly after and administered my shot. I was in the bathroom when my Mother and sister arrived. When I came out of the bathroom, they were shocked to see me walking with a cane, with no assistance. In the back of my mind, I knew I was supposed to have someone there for support, and I expressed that to them. We talked for a few minutes and then took the elevator to the third-floor conference room. I asked my sister to hold on to my arm for effect, so I wouldn't get into trouble.

We were the first to arrive; the social worker, both therapists, the doctor, and the head nurse entered shortly after. The doctor started the meeting by informing the team that all of my blood work had come back negative. The physical therapist spoke next, giving an analysis of my progress:

- I had made numerous gains.
- My balance had improved, with still occasional loss of balance.
- I was able to transfer from my bed to the chair.
- I would receive a new, less restrictive brace soon.
- I could use the base claw cane but only with close supervision.
- I could walk up and down stairs but only if there was someone else with me.
- I was doing a little better making turns.

In regard to my leg,

- My hip muscles were back.
- The muscles to turn were still weak.
- My hamstrings were just starting to come back.
- I had no movement in the ankle, which was typical.

She recommended *possibly* being discharged in two weeks. The goal over that time was to have me walk independently and go up and down stairs. After that, I could receive therapy at home. I mentioned I still couldn't move my toes but hopefully that would happen soon. Dr. Black said that was the key to a complete recovery.

The occupational therapist spoke next. She said she was concerned about my bathing at home. The shower at the rehab was a walk-in, and the one at home was a tub shower, which meant I needed to step up and over to get in. Her recommendation was to use a tub bench for assistance. She said I would probably need help changing the dressing on my head until it was completely healed. Also, I might need help putting my brace on and taking it off, although by the time I left, I would probably have a less restrictive brace that would be easier to manipulate. She agreed with the physical therapist that I could possibly be ready to go home in a couple of weeks.

Then it was time for the head nurse to speak; she stated I was

o   less agitated
o   behaving a little better—locking wheelchair
o   using the bathroom and urinal
o   on Senekot for constipation
o   now tapered to two Decadron
o   constantly being checked for dehydration
o   monitored for blood clots

They all said they were astonished at my progress and optimistic for a complete recovery! They said the next meeting would be on Wednesday, April 21. We all said our goodbyes, and my Mother and sister came back to my room. They both said they were so proud of me and the progress I was making. I said, "What other option did I have?" I thanked them for all their support and assistance and said it would not be impossible but much more difficult to get over this "bump in the road" without family, friends, and medical staff.

Once they left, I was anxious to try my new strengthening exercise without distractions. I closed the door and turned the light off. The television and radio were already off. Then I pulled the shades down. I was ready for the test. Was I totally focused in my prior attempts or, as the physical therapist had said, was I not focused? Soon, we would know if she was correct. I lay facedown on the bed and started the exercise. I pulled my leg up to a ninety-degree angle as instructed and then I very, very slowly let it come to rest back onto the bed; I was expecting it to fall. Without any distractions, on the first try, it moved slowly onto the bed with grace.

I was so overwhelmed I started to sob and realized she was correct. When I initially tried this, I assumed I was totally focused, but I was mistaken. This was the first time in my life I realized how powerful the brain is and how it operates (no pun intended). We all use this complex organ but never really consider how it functions.

I want you to please stop reading this book and look up and focus on only one object. You assume that would be an easy, natural thing to be able to do. What you don't take into consideration is that all the peripheral objects surrounding you come into play. With all these distractions around the focal point, you are never totally focused on one object as I previously believed.

I enthusiastically continued my new and improved exercise for a few hours.

After that, I went outside on my own with my walker because I didn't have permission to walk alone with my cane. It was a brisk but beautiful day, so I stayed outside for about an hour, and when I returned to my room, my dinner had already been delivered. I had a couple of visitors after dinner and was anxious to tell them what I had experienced about the power of the brain. They said they never really thought about it; I said I hadn't either until that day. I found myself much more aware of my surroundings and how I was affected by them. When they left, I continued with my *new* exercise until I fell asleep on top of the bed.

FRIDAY, APRIL 9

I was awakened at 1:00 a.m. for my shot and fell back to sleep. I woke up at 6:00 a.m. excited about the fact that I might be going home in a couple of weeks. I completed my morning routine starting at 7:00 a.m. Now walking with a four-legged cane, I could take a stand-up shower. The nurse said to make sure I walked in with my walker, brought my cane for support, and then held on to the bars. This was another major accomplishment, taking a shower without a walker or wheelchair.

I had combined therapy at 9:00 a.m. They taught me how to get back up if I ever fell; I practiced this exercise for a couple of hours. I had lunch and then purposely fell down so I could try getting up over and over again without the use of a walker. When I was in midstream of falling down, the nurse came in to give me my shot. She rushed over to pick me up before I had the chance to explain that I was just practicing how to get back up if I fell. She exhaled, told me I "scared the daylights" out of her, and then administered my shot. Some friends visited during the day while I was working out. The exercises were strenuous, so I worked up an appetite shortly after eating lunch. I was famished but decided I would just wait for dinner before I ate again.

When the kitchen aide delivered dinner, I told her I was quite hungry and was anxious to see what I was having for dinner. She brought the tray table over, put the food on the table, and said, "Let's see what they prepared for you."

I took the cover off and said, "*Peas!*" The entire dinner consisted of a large bowl of peas and only peas. We both laughed, and I asked if this was a joke.

"Please call the kitchen to find out who the prankster was that sent only peas," I said.

She called the kitchen and apparently my Mother, who had filled out the menu last week, forgot to check off an entree and checked off only a vegetable—peas. Having received my meals for the past week and a half, I knew each meal included an entree, vegetable, and dessert. Instead of calling to see if the menu was filled out properly, the kitchen staff had just sent up peas.

The aide said to them, "It would have made sense to give Mr. Salvo a courtesy call."

I asked, "Could they please send up an entree?"

The aide checked with the kitchen staff who said, "They're all gone; the only other option would be a toasted cheese sandwich."

I said, "That would be fine, but if this happens again, please call me."

We both laughed so hard at this blunder that we were crying. I mentioned how important timing had been during this whole procedure; well, this was imperfect timing. It was the only time I was really starving and the only time I expressed it to the aide. No one was hurt because of this misstep, and we had a good laugh. I received a few phone calls after six, exercised, and fell asleep around nine.

SATURDAY, APRIL 10

I was administered my shot at 1:00 a.m. and fell back to sleep. I completed my morning routine and then a friend of mine came to visit. My sister and Ann came in to visit shortly after and were planning to write in my journal when they noticed I had written in my daily journal. Up until the previous day, a day had not gone by when either my sister or Ann had written about important or mundane events that occurred each day. I thanked them for the daily recordkeeping. I told them that my hand strength had increased enough to give me the ability to write, so I no longer needed assistance. It was not only psychologically helpful, but this exercise would also help improve the mobility in my hand. Their notes, from what I had expressed to them as a daily occurrence as well as what they observed, were very specific. Once I started writing in the journal, my notes were well-defined. I didn't realize the importance until I started writing this book.

As previously mentioned, my sister had given me the journal when I initially entered the rehab facility. She said, "Unless you write the information down, you will never remember the important facts of your recovery."

At the time, my main concern was getting better, not writing in a journal. I never considered how valuable the journal would be, for without the very detailed notes, this book may have never materialized.

My sister brought in a huge box of cards that had been left on my front porch with a note. It was from a colleague of mine who taught English at Kennedy Middle School. Her students made get-well cards, and she delivered them. She was an excellent teacher who, as well as teaching English, taught her students life skills to prepare them for adulthood.

I had lunch, and then neighbors from Cape Cod visited for an hour; I told them it was very thoughtful to make the long journey just to visit me. Once they left, the nurse came in to administer my shot. I worked out that afternoon without any interruptions.

After 6:00 p.m., Father Egan called to tell me he had tried to get in touch with me a few times during the day and didn't get an answer, so he called my Mother who explained I was only taking calls after 6:00 p.m. My great aunt had passed away a couple of days ago. Because I was unable to attend the service, Father Egan, who cocelebrated the service, informed me about the particulars of her funeral. She was very well-known and had numerous friends and family members attend the funeral. Being unable to attend, I sent a floral arrangement.

I had dinner and then another friend came in for a late arrival to watch the Boston Red Sox game with me. He left around nine thirty, and I fell asleep soon after.

SUNDAY, APRIL 11

I was administered my shot at 1:00 a.m. and fell back to sleep. I awoke at 6:30 and completed my usual morning routine. I was going home for the day, so my brother Skip picked me up around 9:00 a.m., and we arrived home at 9:30. At 11:00, the crew started coming: my brothers and their families, relatives and neighbors, Ann, and Father Egan. My Mother made homemade pasta, and did we eat! We had lots of laughs throughout the day. After most of the company left, with help, I walked up to my apartment and paid my bills. Soon I returned and conversed with the few who remained. Ann drove me back to the rehabilitation facility at 7:30; it was a long but enjoyable day. I spoke to my toes at 8:00 p.m. for half an hour with no results and fell asleep at 8:30 p.m.

MONDAY, APRIL 12

I was administered my shot at 1:00 a.m. and fell back to sleep. I woke up at 6:00 a.m. to begin my morning routine. Therapy was at 9:00 with both therapists. We walked outside for a while, and then they demonstrated how to get up if I fell with nothing but a cane to use for assistance. It was much more difficult than I anticipated with only the aid of my four-legged cane and nothing solid to grab on to. The physical therapist told me she would be out the following day and that I would have a substitute for the day. She also mentioned that I would be receiving a new brace, which would cover only my foot and ankle. It would be less restrictive and aid in the continued improvement of my walking skills. It was a brace used on patients for a drop foot, a weakness in the foot caused by trauma.

I had lunch and was administered another shot in the belly. The rest of the day was uneventful, except for the removal of a few meds that were no longer needed. This indicated I was improving because doctors are very cautious about eliminating medications. I had a few visitors, including Ann and my sister, who stayed for about an hour and then left. I went to bed around 9:00 p.m., and at 10:00, I thought I could feel the big toe on my left foot move. I removed the covers to discover I could actually move it. Stunned, I watched it move for about two minutes. Soon after, the other toes followed suit and moved as well. I then let out a yell that may have been heard all the way to the first floor: "*I wiggled my toes ... Hallelujah!*"

The nurse heard me and came running in. She asked, "What happened?"

"I just wiggled my toes ... Hallelujah!" I said.

She sarcastically said, "Wonderful." I was sure she didn't realize the significance.

I said, "Let me explain how important this seemingly insignificant movement is. Dr. Black told me once you can wiggle the toes on your left foot, it means the brain has sent a signal to the furthest part of your body. This could be the first step in achieving a complete recovery."

She said, "Congratulations! You informed me about something I was unaware of."

It was around 10:15 p.m., and except for Ann, I knew everyone would be asleep. I didn't want to frighten them, but I couldn't contain my excitement. I called my Mother, sister, brothers, Ann, Father Egan, and some close friends to tell them the great news: "I wiggled my toes." My family members said that I had frightened them, yet they were aware of what that meant and congratulated me.

When I called some close friends, who like the nurse were obviously unaware of the significance of my toes moving, they responded, "You called me at this time to tell me that?" I then explained to them the importance of this major breakthrough. With each phone call, I got a different reaction, but each conversation ended with a congratulatory response.

I tried but couldn't fall back to sleep and thought it was all the excitement, but there was another factor keeping me awake.

TUESDAY, APRIL 13

I was still awake when the nurse came in to administer my 1:00 a.m. shot.

She said, "I didn't have to wake you tonight. Are you all right?"

I said, "I think so, but I am just having a hard time falling asleep."

She said, "It must have been the excitement about moving your toes."

I only slept for a couple of hours Monday night and was excited about my toes moving, but I was exhausted. I didn't feel well and wasn't sure why. I went through my usual routine and then went back to bed after breakfast. This was the first time I had done this since entering the rehab facility. I called the head nurse and told her I wasn't feeling well. I asked her if she could call the physical and occupational therapists and tell them I would like to cancel for today; she said she would.

Twenty minutes later, a gentleman I had never seen walked in and introduced himself. He told me my physical therapist was out, and he was supposed to work with me for the day. I actually forgot that she would not be working that day. He said the head nurse told him I wanted to skip physical therapy because I wasn't feeling well. I could tell he was upset.

He said, "Last Friday, the physical therapist told me she was going to be out today and asked me if I would be able to cover for her. I was so excited and really looking forward to working with you. The entire staff is talking about you, the *miracle patient*, because of the severity of your case and the strides you have made in such a short time. Is there any chance you could take PT, just for today?"

I said, "Maybe another day, but not today. I am exhausted."

He replied, "This will be my only opportunity to work with you. Could you ... *please?*"

I said, "Sorry, but I really can't."

He was upset and walked out.

I had lunch and then was administered my shot. I had a few visitors during the day and spent most of the day in bed. They all said the same thing: everyone has a bad day once in a while. I said that I wasn't sure why, but I didn't sleep well. A nurse came in with pen and paper to speak to me, but I told her I wasn't having a good day and asked if she would come back another day. She then left and must have mentioned it to the head nurse.

A few minutes later, the head nurse came in to check on me to ask if I was feeling any better. I told her I didn't feel sick, just exhausted, because I only slept a couple hours the night before. I asked her if it could be a reaction to one of the meds that were removed. She mentioned a few, and one was Ativan, which I took for anxiety and to help me sleep. Now it all made sense.

My brother Skip and Ann came in that night and found me in bed. They were concerned, until I told them what had transpired.

The nurse came in around six and gave me my last Decadron—exactly twenty days after the prescription was started. It was such a relief to finish off the prescription drug that had put me into a psychosis. I could now enjoy peace of mind knowing I did not have to worry about a psychotic relapse. I spent almost the entire day in bed and hoped to feel better tomorrow. I fell asleep around 9:00 p.m.

WEDNESDAY, APRIL 14

I woke up at 1:00 a.m. for my shot. The nurse informed me that this would be my last shot.

"Fabulous," I said and then fell back to sleep.

I woke around seven, and I went through my morning routine. At 9:00 a.m., I started with physical therapy. My physical therapist gave me my new brace, which covered only my foot and ankle and was much less restrictive. I went outside, where I walked with my cane; the physical therapist was at my side for safety reasons. I mentioned to her I was feeling poorly yesterday and the reason why.

"Why was the physical therapist so upset when I told him I wasn't up for PT?" I asked.

She said, "Everyone told him how well you were doing, and he was excited about working with you. A number of our patients are older and do not have the stamina. We do have younger patients, but very few are willing to work as hard as you have. We enjoy working with a patient who is progressing at such an accelerated rate."

"Sorry I had to disappoint him, but I really had a bad day."

She said, "Everyone is entitled to a bad day once in a while."

I said, "Maybe another time."

"Yesterday was his last day. Next Monday, he starts another job. That's the reason he said yesterday would be his only chance."

We then went outside, where she wanted me to concentrate on my balance. I am not sure if it was all the rest the day before, but I had great balance, and she was very impressed. I stood on my own by lifting my cane and even shocked myself. After an hour, the physical therapist brought me back inside, and the occupational therapist took over. She wanted to work inside, but I asked if we could please go outside and continue to work on my balance; with some coaxing, she agreed. I was walking with her at my side, and for the first time since my surgery, I felt as if I was really making great gains. I still used my cane as a crutch and pretended to fall a few times, knowing I could recover.

She said, "What are you doing? You're going to get me fired."

"Don't panic. My balance has improved tremendously." After forty-five minutes, she took me inside. She said she was going to have a heart attack if we continued and wouldn't have to worry about being fired.

I had lunch and then continued strengthening my left leg with my new exercise. I believe the increased strength in my left leg allowed me to have more control over my balance and to walk with more confidence. Father Egan visited that afternoon for an hour, and we talked while I was working. Once I rested, we said a few prayers, and he blessed me.

He said, "God is really giving you the strength to persevere."

I said, "He certainly is." The nurse who had been in yesterday returned while he was there.

She said, "I will come back later."

Father Egan said, "I am getting ready to leave." We said our good-byes, and the nurse immediately proceeded to question me about my recovery. I was curious to find out if all these nurses sat down together or if they had a standard questionnaire because they all asked basically the same questions. I didn't want to insult any of them, so I never asked. She stayed for about twenty minutes and then left.

I continued to exercise on the bed and then walked around the room with my cane. I am glad I didn't get caught, because I was supposed to have someone there in case I fell. I think being outside for almost two hours and pushing myself when I worked on my own drained me, because I was exhausted. I thought I should finally be able to sleep through the night without anyone waking me up for my 1:00 a.m. shot. Luckily, for the first time in the last three weeks, I had no visitors after dinner. I watched a little television and fell asleep around 9:00 p.m.

THURSDAY, APRIL 15

Around 1:00 a.m., the door opened, and the nurse turned the light on.

I said, "What are you doing? I thought I was all through with my shot."

She said, "You are, but the head nurse wants to make sure you are breathing."

"Of course I am breathing, but I won't be if you keep bothering me at 1:00 a.m. because you're going to *kill me*."

She said, "Sorry, I just do what I am told."

I said, "I will speak to the head nurse in the morning."

I woke up around 6:30 a.m. to the same routine and then around 7:30 made a call to Ann to wish her a happy fortieth birthday. I walked with my walker to the front desk to talk to the head nurse. I asked her if she would allow me to sleep through the night rather than checking on me to make sure I was *breathing*.

She said, "I want to make sure you're okay."

"I have been here for over two weeks and have had no problems yet, so trust me, I will be okay; you're going to kill me," I responded.

"All right, I will let you sleep. Just don't die on me."

We both laughed.

After speaking to the head nurse, I went back to my room and exercised. Physical therapy started at 9:00 a.m. We worked on walking and turning with my cane and walking up and down stairs. During the morning, I had a few more nurses come in sporadically, one from my floor and two I didn't know. As with everyone else, I answered all their questions. I had lunch and then got back to work.

As I mentioned earlier, I had no visitors the night before, but today was a very different story. My Mother, brother Skip and his family, Ann, a couple of aunts and uncles, a few friends, and two coworkers came in. The entourage started filing in at 1:00 p.m., and everyone left by 8:00. It was a tiring day, so the lights went out around 8:30.

FRIDAY, APRIL 16

Finally, with no 1:00 a.m. shot or nurse checking in on me, I could sleep through the night. I woke up at 6:00 to the same morning routine. Around 9:00, I went to physical and occupational therapy. I continued to walk with a four-legged cane. The physical therapist asked me if I thought I would be able to manage a regular cane; I responded, "Absolutely." She handed me my new walking stick, and we went out to practice all the routine tasks. I did quite well, and both therapists were amazed at my strength, mobility, and balance.

I had a two o'clock appointment with Dr. Jay Loeffler at Mass General Hospital. Ann would be joining me. This was my initial consultation for my upcoming radiation treatment. Ann arrived around 12:30, and she wheeled me outside for the ambulance, which was coming at 12:45. We decided a wheelchair would be much easier to manipulate. The ambulance came on time, and we arrived at the hospital around 1:30. Ann pushed me into the waiting room, and the nurse brought us into his office at 2:00.

Dr. Loeffler arrived a few minutes later, and we exchanged greetings.

He said, "Joe, I called the rehab facility for an update of your progress and they told me you're walking."

I said, "I am taking small steps and have seen improvement each day."

He asked, "Would you be able to walk for me?"

I said, "Sure."

He examined my scar and said, "Hold on a minute." He left the office and returned with his head nurse. He introduced Ann and me to his head nurse.

"Joe, please do your best and try to walk," he said.

At that time, all I could think of was Jesus telling the crippled man to *rise and walk*. Ann was directly behind me for moral and physical support. I knew this would be a daunting task; up until then, I had always used at least a cane for both physical and mental support. I would compare it to driving alone for the first time, which I still remember. When you're learning to drive with your permit or when you just receive your license, there's always someone in the car with you. The first few times you're alone behind the wheel, to whom would you look for support?

The time had come, so I locked the wheelchair, individually raised my foot supports, and then stood up, using my hands against the wheelchair for assistance. I took my first step with my right leg, and it was a little shaky and weak because I had been sitting for quite a while. Once I knew my right leg was firmly planted in front of me, I carefully stepped with my left. I walked about eight feet, reached the wall, turned around, and walked back to the wheelchair, one small step at a time. I walked for the first time without any assistance or cane to lean on if needed; I was a little nervous, but my balance was fine. It took about twenty seconds, which was a long time for that short of a distance, but I did it. Ann and I looked at each other in amazement.

Dr. Loeffler then turned to his nurse and with a bewildered look said, "You have just witnessed a *miracle*. Joe had major surgery just a little over three weeks ago for the removal of a huge tumor. For him to be able to walk at this stage of his recovery should be *medically and physically impossible.* Joe, I am not sure what you've done to get to this point, but continue with your effort. I am still in shock. I have not had the chance to congratulate many patients before they receive radiation."

I said, "In regard to the surgery, it was major, major surgery," and then explained that statement. "Thank you for your kind words, but this was attained by tenacious work."

Now that I was back in my wheelchair, the doctor then asked Ann and me to follow him. We entered a large, bright room. I immediately noticed an eight-foot-long by three-foot-wide table with an enormous machine overhead.

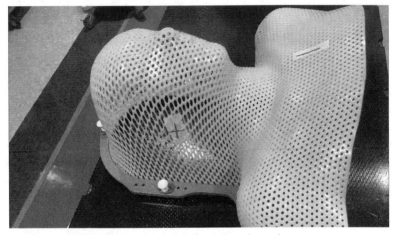

Radiation mask identical to what the author wore.

He said, "You'll have to be fitted for a mask, which will map out the exact points the machine will radiate. When you come for radiation, you will lie on your back, and the mask will be placed over your face and locked into position with six bolts. It is relatively tight to ensure your head is completely immobile. We'll determine the points to be radiated from the MRI, and then the machine will rotate around your head as you remain still on the table. You will have radiation five days a week for six weeks. The average daily treatment will only be fifteen minutes."

He then measured my head and wrote down the readings. He asked if we had any questions. Never having gone through anything like this before, I did some research on radiation. I found out radiation affects everyone differently depending upon the size of the person and the body part being radiated.

As well as this being a book about my experience, I would also like individuals who read it to use it as a surgical and postsurgical guide if needed.

I asked Dr. Loeffler the following questions. They may be of interest to you, the reader, if you need radiation:

o   Are there different strengths of radiation?
    Different doses not strengths.

o   Are there any dietary restrictions?
    Rarely—almost never

o   Will I need another MRI?
    Yes—usually every year until year five, and then every two to three years

o   Are there any medications you should avoid when being radiated?
    No

o   Will the effects of radiation always set you back (tired, lethargic, and so on)?
    Yes—but to a varying degree—sometimes barely, sometimes enough so that you will want to take a nap every day

I thanked him, and we said our goodbyes and left.

When he described my ability to walk as a miracle, it didn't really make an impact on me because I was just doing what had to be done in order to recover. From everything I was told, without all my hard work and tenacity, I possibly would have never walked again. I mentioned to other medical professionals that Dr. Loeffler was my radiologist. They all agreed that he was one of the best if not the best brain radiologist in the world. As I look back, his statement has more of an impact on me now than it did then. For a man of his stature to take the time to summon his nurse and then make that comment leads me to believe I must have been doing something special.

Ann and I took the ambulance back to the rehab facility and arrived around 4:30 p.m. She stayed for a few minutes and then left. I had dinner and then worked out on my new exercise until company arrived. Now, whenever I exercised, I asked for silence and needed darkness in the room. I explained to visitors the reasoning behind that. They understood, although they were somewhat skeptical. I went to bed early after everyone left.

SATURDAY, APRIL 17

I had the same morning routine and then continued to exercise. Once lunch arrived, I told the aide to tell the kitchen I wouldn't be there for dinner. The physical therapist was out for the day. The occupational therapist was unable to work with me in the morning, so I had occupational therapy for two hours that afternoon. Occupational therapy now overlapped with physical therapy, because the occupational therapist realized I was able to perform tasks that she originally stated I shouldn't have been capable of accomplishing for years, if ever. To be kind, I never mentioned it to her, but I do remember reflecting about what I had attained in such a short period of time. Two and a half weeks prior, she was showing me how to pour a glass of orange juice from a wheelchair.

She came to my room shortly after lunch. I told her about my day on Friday and how I walked without any assistance, wearing merely my brace. She was astonished and congratulated me but said to make sure I had something to hold on to in case I needed it. She was always cautious about any advancement I made. I said that Ann was right behind me, but I never required her assistance. We started inside and worked for half an hour, and then I asked if we could work outside. She said we could as long as I promised not to pretend to fall; I agreed. We worked on going up and down the curb for about half an hour and then walked around the building a few times. Once I finished, I returned to my room to exercise on my own. When finished, I asked the nurse if I could take another shower. I was going out later that day and had been perspiring. She said that wouldn't be a problem, just to be sure to bring in my walker in case I lost my balance. I was able to take care of myself without any assistance, and it felt good to be independent again.

I was ready at four o'clock and then relaxed until Skip picked me up at five. We headed to Vinny Testa's for an Italian meal to celebrate Ann's fortieth birthday. My entire family, Ann, and an aunt and uncle were there to join us in the celebration. This was my first time dining in a restaurant postsurgery. I intentionally avoided mentioning the "miracle" at Dr. Loeffler's office when I spoke to any family members, because I wanted Ann to tell the story. I said grace and thanked family and friends for all the support and blessings they had bestowed upon me over the past three weeks. I wished Ann a happy birthday and said, "Ann has a story to share with you before we eat."

She proceeded to describe everything that took place in Dr. Loeffler's office, from calling in his nurse, to knowing I had been taking steps, and then asking me to walk. "Without any assistance," she said, "Joe lifted himself up from the wheelchair, walked about eight feet, turned around, and went back and sat down. Dr. Loeffler stated to his nurse that she had witnessed a miracle." After a round of applause followed by a few tears, all agreed that it was truly a miracle.

We had a joyous time and now with good reason, a lot of laughs indeed. After dinner, we said our goodbyes, kissed each other, and went back to our respective homes. Skip took me back to the rehab facility. I watched a little television, exercised my left arm, and said my prayers, and lights went out around nine.

SUNDAY, APRIL 18

I was going home for the day, so after breakfast, I worked out before my shower. I showered on my own and forgot to inform the nurse; nothing was said. My sister, Patty, picked me up at 9:15 a.m. She signed me out, and we headed home.

I spent some time with my Mother and then carefully walked up to my apartment. They were still worried that I might fall, so whenever I went up or down the stairs, someone was there to watch me. After a while, I came back down on my own (even though they said to let them know when I was coming back down so they could watch me). I am stubborn and knew I could walk safely down on my own.

My sister and I then went outside and walked around the block. I felt confident walking with my cane and occasionally walked just holding it off the ground for safety reasons. When we returned home, I was getting tired and had to sit down. That was a lot of exercise and the longest walk I had taken with a cane. I sat for a little while and then joined my Mother and Patty for a five-minute drive to Skip's house for lunch; Ann and my niece joined us. There was not the usual crew because we had all been together the previous night.

After lunch, a few of us took a short walk outside to work off the pasta, even though most of us had eaten pasta last night. Italians can never have enough pasta. My walk was really short because I was exhausted from the walk I had taken earlier. Then we sat down and shared stories about the past few weeks and how all our lives had changed. It's strange how life can be going along so smoothly, and then, all of a sudden, your world is turned upside down. But you learn to deal with it; many times, you have no choice. After a few hours of storytelling, we had a light dinner. Being Italian, most of what we do revolves around food. After dinner, we said our goodbyes, and around seven o'clock, Ann drove me back to the rehabilitation facility and then left. I signed back in, went back to my room, and sat up for a while. It was a tiring day, so around eight thirty, I said my prayers and went to bed.

CHAPTER 9
MY LAST WEEK AT WINGATE AT BRIGHTON

MONDAY, APRIL 19 (PATRIOT'S DAY)

I had the same morning routine. The physical therapist and occupational therapist worked together simultaneously. The physical therapist was out on Saturday, so I thought she may have been unaware of what occurred at my appointment with Dr. Loeffler. They both arrived in my room around 9:00 a.m. I told the physical therapist that I had a story that I wanted to share with her. I told her about my appointment and how he was amazed at my ability to walk, considering I had had major surgery slightly over three weeks ago. He called it a *miracle*.

She said, "You are a miracle. You have progressed more than any patient we have had, in such a short period of time. Actually, the occupational therapist already told me what took place in Dr. Loeffler's office, but you looked so enthusiastic about telling me that I didn't want to spoil the excitement. At this point, most patients are in a wheelchair, many are using a walker, and very few have a cane or brace."

I told her, "Last week, I spoke to one patient who has returned for therapy every few months for the past ten years. He also had a meningioma tumor same as I and had it removed through surgery. His tumor was much smaller than mine. He's eight years younger than I and still in a wheelchair. I asked him why he was unable to walk.

"His response was, 'This should never have happened to me.'"

I said, "It's not fair for anyone to have to undergo major surgery, but you have to work and fight to enjoy the life you led prior to the surgery. He had surgery ten years ago and is still in a wheelchair. It's just ridiculous."

They both agreed and said, "We know whom you're talking about. He was never willing to devote any time to his recovery. He felt sorry for himself and, instead of working, just sat in his wheelchair and cried."

"I worked less than a month, and I am walking again. I wasn't about to spend the rest of my life in a wheelchair. I knew with my strong belief in God, Dr. Black as my surgeon, support from family and friends, and assistance from staff like yourself I would walk. What's up for today?"

First, I had occupational therapy. She had me walk outside with my cane and then practice getting up without the use of a cane. After an hour, the physical therapist took over and said, "Let's head back to your room." I thought that was unusual, because I never had physical therapy in my room.

The three of us took the elevator up to the second floor, and on the way up, the physical therapist shocked me and said, "Are you ready to walk without any supportive device to lean on?"

While I am writing this, it's still emotional, and I have shed a few tears thinking about what I had accomplished in less than four weeks.

I said, "Absolutely."

"Once we get off the elevator, I want you to hand me your cane, and without assistance, staying close to the wall, walk back to your room."

I was a little nervous but knew it could be accomplished because at home I had walked without using a cane but held it for moral support. When we walked out of the elevator, the physical therapist asked me for my cane. I handed her my cane and looked down the hall to my room. It was only about eighty feet, but I felt as if I were preparing to run the Boston Marathon.

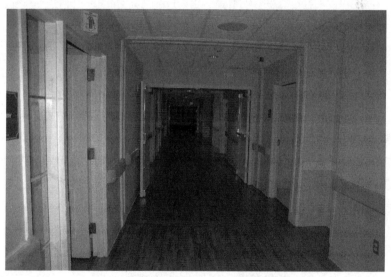

Hall from elevator to author's destination –
room 110. My Boston Marathon.

I started down the hall, taking one small step at a time. I always made sure my right foot was firmly planted on the ground before taking a step with my left foot. I lost my balance slightly, but in retrospect, I think it was more nerves than lack of balance. As I walked by the nursing station, the head nurse looked up, shook her head in astonishment and said, "I am amazed."

In approximately three minutes, I proudly walked from the elevator to my room. Once I made it to my room, they all clapped and congratulated me. It was very emotional, and we all shed a few tears of joy. At this point, it was like *winning* the Boston Marathon. Runners are oblivious of their accomplishments, until they cross the finish line. At that moment, all their emotions emerge.

Now with complete confidence and better stability, I walked back and forth from the elevator to my room a few more times. The therapists told me my gait looked stable but to continue to walk near the wall for support. Both therapists again congratulated me. I thanked them for all their physical and emotional support.

The physical therapist said we had a meeting scheduled for Wednesday afternoon at two. A number of the staff would be present, as well as any members of my family and friends who would like to attend. After physical therapy, I went to my room and immediately called everyone who took part in my recovery. I told them of my accomplishment: walking without any supportive device, just a small brace. Because it was a holiday, many were home, and for the rest, I left messages. Lunch had been delivered an hour earlier, but I was too excited to eat and had to tell everyone what had transpired.

Early that afternoon, I watched the Boston Red Sox and Boston Marathon, while continually stretching my leg. Knowing I had the ability to walk, I was more motivated than ever to continue to improve. I continued exercising for the rest of the afternoon. I ate dinner, and then my brother Skip, Ann, and a few relatives were kind enough to visit, even though we had been together the past two days. They were excited about my being able to walk. They all left around eight. I called friends and relatives I didn't reach that afternoon to tell them about my major breakthrough. I said my prayers and went to bed at nine thirty. It took a while for me to fall asleep because of all the excitement during the day.

TUESDAY, APRIL 20

I woke up around five thirty and performed the same routine starting at seven. I went to occupational therapy at nine. My therapist was ecstatic I was able to walk without any assistance. She asked if I would like to walk outside. I said, "Positively." This was as big a step for her as it was for me because she was very conservative and normally allowed the physical therapist to have me take the next step (literally and figuratively). The physical therapist was out for the day, so she must have spoken to her about what to work on.

We always took the elevator, but I told her I would prefer to walk down the stairs. For the past three plus weeks, I had been unable to use stairs but now had the ability to do so. Through this whole process, I would continually reflect on what life was like one month earlier. Once outside, without any aid but my brace, I walked around the rehabilitation facility. She was always nearby for support, but I never needed any help. Even *I* was surprised with my balance and walking ability; we continued for twenty minutes.

She said, "Now I want you to walk up and down the curb. Do you remember the saying?"

I said, "I do, 'You left to go down to hell, but you go right up to heaven.'"

She said, "Close enough."

I practiced that for twenty minutes. It sounds easy, but every time I went up or down, I had to recall the saying: "You left to go down to hell, but you go right up to heaven." After repeatedly walking up and down curbs for so many years, it was weird to have to think about which foot to lead with. After a while, it became much easier.

She said, "When you walk around the inside of the building, you can walk without the use of a cane, but continue to walk close to the wall for support. If you walk outside, take your cane or make sure someone is with you, even though you know how to get up if you fall."

On my way back to my room, I looked at the bulletin board next to the elevator, which displayed the daily activities. Because of my grueling schedule, I had never participated in any activities run by the nursing facility. With no physical therapy that afternoon, I had some extra time. At two o'clock in the conference room, a nun was scheduled to lead the Rosary. With all the blessings I had received over the past month, I decided I would pray the Rosary as a thank-you to God. I had lunch, worked out for a little while, and then just before two walked up to the conference room with only my brace on. It felt strange because I had now walked totally alone, no cane or aid to assist me. It felt like the first time I drove alone; there was no one there for support. I made it to the room without incident. There were about ten other patients there. Shortly after two, the nun walked in and introduced herself. She passed out a few books explaining how to pray the Rosary. We all prayed the Rosary, and when finished, we thanked her, and she left.

I returned to my room, and a short time later, Father Egan arrived for a visit. I told him I had prayed the Rosary a little earlier; he said it was a kind gesture. I said it was the least I could do considering the grace God had bestowed upon me since my surgery; he agreed and gave me a blessing. He said he was very impressed with my progress. He frequently spoke with my family members and was kept informed of my improvement but knew it would take a while for a complete recovery. He stayed for another hour and then left. The rest of the afternoon and evening were quiet. After dinner, I watched a little television, said my prayers, and went to bed.

WEDNESDAY, APRIL 21

Same morning routine. The staff of Wingate decided a couple of days ago that we should have a meeting to discuss my future. I was excited because two weeks before, in our last meeting, it was mentioned that I might go home in a couple of weeks, but nothing was definite. Considering the progress I had made with my ability to walk, I was pretty certain they were sending me home very soon.

At nine, I had occupational therapy. The occupational therapist said, "It's such a beautiful day. Would you like to walk outside?"

I said, "That would be enjoyable."

I walked around the building, up and down the curbs, for an hour with nothing but a small brace on my left leg. Immediately after occupational therapy, I had physical therapy, and we continued with the same exercise. I was exhausted, but for me, it was my Fourth of July, because with the ability to walk on my own, I had gained my independence. I didn't have permission to drive but hoped that would come very soon. I was so proud of myself because in less than a month I had advanced from a wheelchair to a walker to a four-legged cane to a cane and now just a short brace, which I knew would soon be removed. I had accomplished something the staff at Wingate, upon my arrival, had stated could not be done. No other patient with a tumor the size of mine had walked out of their rehab facility.

After physical therapy, I relaxed and then had lunch. The meeting was scheduled for two, and my Mother, sister, and Ann arrived around one forty-five. When they came into my room, they could tell I was excited about the meeting, because I was grinning from ear to ear. My sister, Patty, said I looked like I was ready to go home.

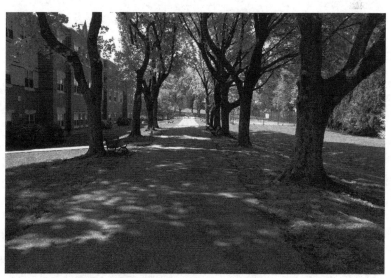

Beautiful day to walk the grounds at Wingate at Brighton.

"Remember what they said at the meeting two weeks ago, that I may be going home in a couple weeks?" I replied. "Well, it's almost two weeks, and I think today they are going to tell me to start packing."

Ann said, "You really have progressed beyond everyone's expectations."

We continued our conversation until the nurse came in to tell us the meeting would be starting shortly in the conference room. We walked up, entered the conference room, and were greeted by the doctor, occupational therapist, physical therapist, head nurse, one of my personal nurses, and the social worker.

We all knew each other, so we simply shook hands. I don't recall the exact order, but each staff member spoke and said how proud he or she was of me and my determination to walk.

I said, "I did what was necessary for me to have some quality in my life. From my perspective there was no option; I either work and walk or feel sorry for myself and remain in that wheelchair or use a walker for the rest of my life. I can tell you that with a strong belief in God and the assistance of family, friends, medical staff, and Dr. Black, it was a much easier challenge to overcome. So, when am I going home?"

The head nurse responded, "Friday morning."

"*Thank You, God!* I want to thank each one of you for helping me get over this little bump in the road. I know there were times when I was difficult to deal with, so thank you for putting up with me."

They said I did have my moments, but it was inspiring to watch me progress these past three plus weeks. One of them interjected that it was like bringing up a child and watching him or her grow through the years; only this was a much more condensed version. Now that I knew I was leaving, they all wanted to reiterate what they had already said.

The doctor said, "You have progressed beyond what anyone believed could be accomplished. You will continue to receive physical therapy at home or in an outpatient facility. You have to be very careful; don't be too daring. Use the cane if needed, and try to walk in areas where there is something to grab onto. One mishap and you could end up back in the rehab facility."

I said, "I will be very careful and not take any unnecessary chances."

My Mother said, "Don't worry; we'll watch him and be at his side for support."

The head nurse said, "As I have told you in the past, you are a 'miracle.' You really have succeeded beyond anyone's expectations. I wish you the best of luck in whatever your challenge is and hope to see you run the Boston Marathon someday."

The physical therapist said, "It was a pleasure to work with you and watch you grow this past month. As I mentioned to you, most of our patients are elderly and can't and don't improve as you have."

The occupational therapist said, "You proved me wrong. You said you would walk out of this rehab facility, and I said it has never happened, but, thankfully, I was wrong."

My personal nurse said, "It was a pleasure working with you. It's nice to see a continuous smile on a patient, and you certainly did radiate that room with your smile."

I thanked them for their kind words; we all said our goodbyes, and the four of us headed back to my room.

When we arrived back in room 110, I said, "Finally, I am going home." My Mother, sister, and Ann said it was nice to hear all those kind words from the staff. I agreed, considering the medical staff as well as family and friends were all so important to my recovery and equally responsible for helping me get my life back. We all became emotional. We said our goodbyes, and they left.

I spent the rest of the afternoon working out and calling family and friends to give them the good news. I had dinner delivered and told the aide to cancel all my meals after Friday morning because I was going home. She said she knew and congratulated me. I watched some television without any visitors because everyone knew I would be home in a couple of days. I turned the television off around nine and said my prayers but did not fall asleep until eleven.

I was psyched.

THURSDAY, APRIL 22

After following the same morning routine, I went to a concurrent occupational and physical therapy for the last time at Wingate at Brighton. The three of us walked around the building and talked about how much I had improved since entering the rehab facility. They agreed and said not every patient had such a happy ending to an unfortunate circumstance.

They both said, "Once you settle down and accomplish your goal of walking completely on your own, even without that brace, you must write a book."

I told them, "Once I find the time, I will write my book."

I thanked them for all they had done, we said our goodbyes, and I *walked* back to my room. I continued to work out and then had my last lunch at Wingate at Brighton.

I worked out through the afternoon, without any visitors. I had dinner, and then, shortly after, my brother Skip and a few other friends and relatives came in, even though it was my last night. I continued to exercise between visitors, and they were all happy for me, because they knew that this was my last night in the rehab facility. I said my prayers and then went to bed around nine with a smile on my face. I was appreciative for all the staff had done but, as you can imagine, very anxious to go home.

FRIDAY, APRIL 23

I woke up around five and packed my clothes, get-well cards, and pills. I took a shower, shaved, and then had breakfast at seven. The head nurse came in around eight to go over my medication. She gave me the phone number of my case manager to arrange for physical therapy at home.

She said, "It may be a while down the road, but you have to write a book. You could be an inspiration to other patients in your condition. We can no longer tell anyone in your condition, when you entered the rehab, that they won't be able to walk out of here."

I said, "Once my life is back to normal, I will write a book."

I was leaving at 9:00 a.m. and waited around for a few minutes. My brother-in-law and niece had arrived, and I was ready to leave but said to myself, "What am I forgetting?" Then it came to me. I asked my brother-in-law to please wait a few minutes; I had one last task that I had to complete. I *walked* down the hall, *walked* down the stairs to the first floor, and headed toward the occupational therapist's office. I peeked in, and she was at her desk doing paperwork. I *walked* to the kitchen we used for occupational therapy. There was no one in the room, so I entered, opened the cabinet, and took out a glass. I opened the refrigerator, grabbed the orange juice, and proudly poured it into the glass. I went to the occupational therapist's office and knocked on the door. She told me to come in. I entered the room with a huge smile, *walked* over to her desk, and placed the glass of orange juice on her desk.

I said, "This is the glass of orange juice I promised to *walk* into your office and place on your desk before I left here."

We looked at each other, gave each other a hug, and teared up as if an enormous weight had been lifted. She made the same statement as the head nurse.

"Never again can I tell anyone who is in the condition you were when you arrived that they won't walk out of here," she said.

Hearing this again made me realize I had done something very special. We said our goodbyes, and I headed back to my room.

A couple of my nurses were waiting for me. We hugged, and I told them I would be back to visit; they wished me well and left. I walked up to the head nurses' station with only the use of a small brace.

I said, "This is not a final goodbye. I will be back to visit."

She said, "It's too bad you have to leave on such a rainy day." It was absolutely pouring.

"I don't see any rain; for me, it's all sunshine."

She said, "I see your attitude hasn't changed."

"It never will."

"Your last official duty is to sign this discharge form, which states the reason for your discharge. It reads, 'Your health has improved sufficiently so that you no longer need the services provided by the nursing facility.' I never thought you would be signing this form, with this statement, in less than a month. I will tell you again, what you accomplished, in a little over three weeks, may have been a lot of work, but I look at this as a *miracle*. You have changed the protocol of the rehabilitation facility."

I said, "Thank you for all you have done, and I promise to come back to visit."

She said, "Don't forget to write that book. Other patients must know that this goal can be attained."

"Someday I will write a book, and hopefully it will help others who are in a similar situation I was in."

I continued walking out and stopped to thank the operator/secretary for all she had done. We gave each other a hug. She sarcastically told me that, although she enjoyed my being there, it was great to see me leave because her job had increased twofold, with all the get-well cards I had received. We laughed and gave each other another hug, and I left.

As gratifying as it was to leave the rehab facility, it was still emotional. I had been there for twenty-four days, and the staff had been a huge part of my life. Whether or not I agreed with everything they did or said, they performed their duties to the best of their ability.

They were committed to my progress, and eventual recovery, and for that, I am forever grateful.

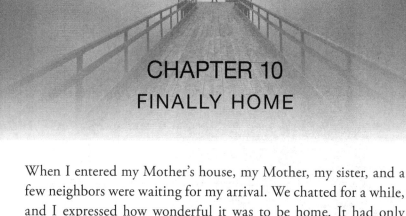

CHAPTER 10
FINALLY HOME

When I entered my Mother's house, my Mother, my sister, and a few neighbors were waiting for my arrival. We chatted for a while, and I expressed how wonderful it was to be home. It had only been a month since my surgery, but it seemed like an eternity. I told them that I could have overcome this *bump on the road* on my own if I had had to, but it would have been much more difficult to accomplish without my strong belief in God and the assistance, support, and prayers from family and friends and the entire medical staff, especially Dr. Black. It was great to have all the questions and unknowns in the past, and I was looking forward to the future.

After an hour, I thanked them all, gave them a kiss, and headed up to my apartment to rest.

My Mother said, "Now be careful," as she watched me walk up the stairs to make sure I didn't fall. "Tomorrow we will go shopping and buy you some food."

I replied, "I am not sure what I will buy for food, but I am definitely buying some orange juice."

She was aware of what I was referring to, so we both laughed. I still didn't have permission to drive, so I would have to rely on others for any errands.

It was great to be home in my own apartment and for the first time in a month sleep in my own bed. I made some phone calls to set up physical therapy at home. I had lunch with my Mother and then worked out in my apartment during the afternoon. My brother Skip picked up my Mother and me and brought us to his house for dinner. I can't remember what we ate, but there must have been some pasta somewhere in the meal. He brought us home around eight. I gave my Mother a kiss and headed up to my apartment. I reflected on what had transpired the past month and then, totally exhausted, said my prayers and went to bed.

SATURDAY, APRIL 24

I slept very well, woke up around six, and completed my morning exercises. I showered and shaved, and, not having any food in the apartment, went to my Mother's for breakfast. She said that we would leave to go shopping around nine.

We shopped and bought enough food for at least two weeks so as not to burden anyone next week. My walking had greatly improved, but I was a little apprehensive about carrying the bags of groceries into the house, although I didn't mention it to my Mom.

Once we arrived home, my Mother got out of the car, brought in a bag of groceries, and then looked at me as I stood by the car. She said, "Hurry up with the rest of the bags; some of the items have to go into your refrigerator and freezer."

I laughed and then brought them in without a problem. This was when I realized everything was back to normal. Because of my Father's disability, my Mother was always in charge and would *bark* out orders. The previous day, she was worried about me walking around the house. Just one day later, she had confidence that I could not only walk without assistance but carry in the groceries.

That was my Mom, and it was great to hear.

SUNDAY, APRIL 25

I woke up early and completed my morning routine. I then attended the nine o'clock Mass with my brother Skip. Mass was at Sacred Heart Church, where Father Egan was pastor, although he was not offering that particular Mass. Sacred Heart was the Church where I was baptized, made my First Communion, and was confirmed. Because it was a neighborhood church in an Italian section of the city, I knew quite a few people. After Mass, about twenty people, some of whom I had been in touch with throughout this process and some who told me they followed my progress, said they were glad to see me. They were all shocked to see how well I was doing because they had spoken to family or friends about the severity of the operation and realized the chance of my walking in the near future was improbable.

I said, "You know how strong-willed and stubborn I am. Once they told me it would take years before I could walk, I had to prove them wrong." After we had talked for a few minutes and I had explained to them what I had been through, we left. Skip brought me home, and I spent the rest of the day relaxing and exercising.

It was great to be home.

MONDAY, APRIL 26

The day was routine, although I did undergo another MRI. As mentioned prior, they placed a helmet over my head with a mirror that was angled to see out the MRI tube. For me, it helped just being able to see out of the tube. With all the MRIs I had had to this point, I had never had to press the bulb they place in your hand to signal a problem. Once in the tube, I realized there was no mirror on the helmet to see out. I started to hyperventilate and pressed the bulb.

The technician came from behind his desk in the scan room, entered the room where the MRI was taking place, pushed the switch to remove me from the tube, and asked what was wrong.

I said, "I am not comfortable without a mirror to see out of the tube."

He said, "When we removed the helmet from our last patient, the mirror broke off. We have no other helmet available at this time."

I told him, "I am not sure I can complete the test without a mirror."

He said, "Well, let me try something. The mirror is still intact." He took a piece of *gum* out of his mouth and stuck it on the back of the mirror and then placed it on the helmet. He angled it to my satisfaction and slid me back into the MRI tube. All I could think of now was the mirror falling off onto my face.

He said, "How's that?"

"Perfect."

We both laughed, and he completed the test. That was the only time I ever had to press the bulb—never before and never after. While in the tube, the only thing that kept me from laughing hysterically was the fact that I would have had to redo the scan.

I thought to myself, *we have a multimillion-dollar machine, and we need a piece of gum to make it work properly.*

TUESDAY, APRIL 27

I completed my morning routine. At 9:00 a.m., my first outpatient home physical therapist arrived. With relentless exercising on my own, even my left leg had gained back most of its strength. I was still having slight difficulty with my balance. The physical therapist said, because of my ability to walk as well as I was, I would need a physical therapist whose skill level was more advanced in working with patients who had balance issues.

Being a teacher, my thoughts were, *just one lesson and I graduated to the next class.*

I thanked her and said that would be helpful because my principal problem at that time was my balance. She said she would have the other physical therapist contact me and left. Up until then, I never realized physical therapists had specific skill levels. The rest of the day was routine, as I worked out and completed daily activities.

Starting that Thursday, I would require thirty-three radiation treatments, every weekday at 10:00 a.m. I still didn't have permission to drive, so I needed someone to take me to Mass General. That afternoon, I made a number of calls to family and friends who had offered their services. I set up a schedule for the first two weeks. Many offered to drive in the future, so I set up a schedule for the following weeks. After only a few more phone calls, my treatment calendar was complete.

WEDNESDAY, APRIL 28

I woke up, and I no longer needed the small brace. Because of all my work and exercise, my walking was continually improving. I still had a slight problem with my gait, but that was due to the tumor still attached to the nerve controlling my left side. Hopefully, the radiation would someday remove the residual tumor.

After having progressed through a wheelchair, a walker, a four-legged cane, and a regular cane, I now would also never require the use of a brace again.

CHAPTER 11
MY LIFE HAS CHANGED,
BUT I AM WALKING!

THURSDAY, APRIL 29

I woke up at 5:30 a.m. and was anxious to find out about what radiation entailed, even though Dr. Loeffler explained what would take place. One of my aunts picked me up at 8:30 a.m. We left very early because, being the first day, neither one of us knew about the parking situation. The streets along the route were congested, so thankfully we had given ourselves enough time. We arrived at 9:30 a.m. for my ten o'clock appointment.

My aunt dropped me off in front of Mass General Hospital and parked the car. I was early and found the doctor's office. Needless to say, I filled out some paperwork, gave it to the secretary, and was told to wait for the nurse to bring me to the radiation room. My aunt had arrived in the office shortly after.

Just a few minutes before 10:00 a.m., the nurse came and brought me in for radiation. It was the same room I had been in when being mapped. The nurse had me lie on my back on the table and place my head in an exact location to properly align with the mask. She then brought out a mask with my name on it. It contained numerous pinholes for breathing.

She said, "This will be screwed into place and worn during the radiation."

I said, "It doesn't look very comfortable; how will I breathe?"

"It's very restricting, but you will only be on the machine for approximately fifteen minutes. In order to radiate the proper area, it has to be tight. The pinholes will allow you to breathe."

I said, "Thankfully it's only for fifteen minutes."

She then arranged the mask directly over my face and, with six screws, locked it into position. It was difficult to breathe, and the mask was extremely confining, but there was no other alternative. The doctor and nurse confirmed the alignment and then left the room.

The radiation machine released a low sound as I was being radiated. It remained in one spot for a period of time and then would rotate to another position. It indeed did take only fifteen minutes, but it seemed so much longer because of the situation.

For the next thirty-two days, not including weekends, a friend or relative would drive me to Mass General every morning for a 10:00 a.m. appointment. The last two weeks of radiation, I was sleeping about fifteen hours a day. I mentioned that to the nurse, and she said that was normal. Two weeks after I finished my treatments, the effects of the radiation began to wear off, and I started to regain my energy.

Before I left Wingate, the physical therapist gave me a list of exercises to work on at home.

Most of my exercises consisted of stretching, regaining my balance, and strengthening my left leg.

I would do the following:
- toss and catch a large ball in the air with a ball behind my head against a wall (balance)
- push-ups (strength)
- small stool—stepping up on a stool and over, also sidestep up and over

- squats standing on a pillow (balance)
- elastic band—work the knee and ankle back and forth
- chair—while sitting, lift myself up without holding on (strength)
- standing in place—heel raises (strength)
- knees to chest (stretching)
- sitting down, bring knees to chest and rotate to the right and left (stretch)
- lying on back—raise left leg up and stretch over my body

It wasn't always easy, and occasionally, there were times when I would struggle, but when I became discouraged, I would think about how far I had come. Many times, I would revisit the first time I had occupational therapy and her statement to me about why she was teaching me how to pour a glass of orange juice. *"If you want to live by yourself, these are the things you will have to learn. If you want any quality of life, for possibly the rest of your life, this is how you will live."* After recalling her statement, I would work even harder.

For the next month following radiation, I had physical therapy three times a week in various offices, Winchester Hospital, and my home. My gait when I walked was still somewhat problematic, but what was key was that I *walked*.

I was given permission to drive three months after being released from Wingate. It was very emotional, and I recalled sitting in the wheelchair in the front of Wingate questioning whether or not I would ever drive again. Whenever I parked my car in a lot, I purposely parked away from my destination for exercise. I still had a slight limp and minor problems walking up and down the curb, but I never applied for a handicap card. I thought that others who were less fortunate could use the handicap space.

To show my appreciation, sometime that month, I purchased and delivered gold bracelets for the staff at Wingate as well as Dr. Black's nurses Donna DelloIacono and Nancy Olsen Bailey. I was told by one of his nurses that Dr. Black was interested in models, so I purchased a Boston Lighthouse model and gave it to him.

Five years postsurgery, I threw a thank-you party for approximately seventy family and friends who were the most significant in my recovery.

CHAPTER 12
THOUGHTS OF FAMILY AND FRIENDS

During surgery and postsurgery, I was so concerned about the operation and then recovery that I never considered the anguish others must have been enduring. Because we are such a close family, I couldn't imagine the extent of anxiety they had experienced during my surgery. What was supposed to be an eight-hour operation, through the fault of no one, took twelve hours to complete. For over a month, the members of my immediate family as well as some close friends, had focused their attention on my well-being. Their lives had been altered in order to support me physically and emotionally during my ordeal.

While recovering, I occasionally did ask them to share their feelings about what was taking place. I recorded some of what they said, but before writing this book, I interviewed them to see if their thoughts had changed now that they had had time to reflect. What follows in this chapter is a combination of what I had asked while recovering as well as my current interviews. I asked the following questions of my immediate family and my friend Ann. I intertwined the thoughts, in their exact words, of my Mother; my brothers,

Skip and Chris; and Ann. My sister, Patty, offered to write her own thoughts, which I have included verbatim.

During my youth in the late 1950s and through most of the 1960s, it was commonly believed that if someone developed cancer or a brain tumor, he or she didn't have much time to live. I asked my family and Ann what their thoughts were when they heard I had a brain tumor.

My Mom said, "I didn't know what to think. I just kept saying as a family we had been through so much, and now this has to happen." She was primarily referring to my Dad, who had been sick almost all of their married life and thus had required a great deal of care as his health deteriorated.

My brother Skip said, "I wasn't overly concerned about the outcome as long as you had a great doctor." He soon discovered that I had Dr. Black, the *best in the world.*

My brother Chris's first thought was "Whether or not it was operable." Once he found out it was, he said he became more relieved.

Ann said, "I could not believe my ears when you told me. How could it happen to someone so young and healthy? Just goes to prove that we can never take life or our health for granted. At the time I told you that you could rely on us for whatever you need, whatever we can do to get you back on your feet."

I asked them if they ever thought I wouldn't make it. My Mom's major concern was her lack of knowledge about a brain tumor. "I was kind of frightened and didn't know what to think. I kept praying to God that you would be all right."

Skip said, "Because of the doctor, I had no doubt you would make it."

Chris said, "I wasn't sure because I didn't know the circumstances."

Ann said, "I never had a moment of doubt. Your zest for life, your family, and your perseverance is a recipe that can't be beat."

My Mother, Patty and her husband, Skip, and Ann were all in the waiting room during the surgery. I never thought to ask them until a couple of years after the surgery what it was like to sit there and wait without knowing what the outcome would be.

My Mother said, "It was like a bad dream."

My brother Skip said, "We had a lot of fun because we had to, in order to not be nervous."

Ann said, "It seemed like an eternity; twelve hours will do that. There were funny moments. I don't remember any of us leaving the room for food or coffee, because we were concerned we would miss an update. I was worried because it took so long."

I asked what they thought of the process, from the surgery through rehab. My Mom said, "I had all my faith in Dr. Black. I knew he was well known and that he was a great doctor and would get you out of this mess."

Skip and Chris both said, "Other than the psychosis, everything went very well."

Ann said, "It was a little bit of a roller coaster: meeting Dr. Black, the surgery, and finally Wingate. I was worried but knew you were in good hands and were going to be okay. It never crossed my mind that you wouldn't survive, but I was concerned that Wingate was going to be a rehab for old people; indeed, it was not. I think the fact that you were young gave the entire rehab staff an extra special push to get you out of there."

Did you think I would walk again? My Mom said, "I didn't know it would affect your walking as much as it did. I was kind of surprised."

Skip said, "If you thought you could do it, I was convinced you would."

Chris said, "Yes. People fight and beat the thoughts of the medical field."

Ann said, "No matter what you were told, there was no doubt in my mind that you would ever walk again."

I asked Skip what his thoughts were when I called and asked him, "Would you please come in and kill me?"

He said, "I didn't know what to think and only shared the call with Ann and Patty." He realized it would have been too much for my Mom to handle. "I didn't want to worry Chris and his family."

Skip said, "When I called Ann and told her what you said, I broke down and cried."

Ann said, "Complete craziness. That's not you, so I assumed something was amiss with the steroid reaction."

Being in the medical field, she realized it must have had something to do with the steroids, and she shared that with Skip. Both of them agreed that it was very frightening to see me experience a psychosis.

I asked each of them for their final thoughts about the entire process. My Mom said, "I want to thank God that you are all right. The Lord has been good to us, even though we have had our troubles."

Skip said, "I think everything went well. You were in good hands."

Ann said, "There was never a moment that you questioned whether or not you would have a good outcome. In the rehab, you were always doing something. You are a remarkable man to have gone through this, with faith in God, Dr. Black, family, friends, and never a negative moment. Hopefully many more people will benefit from your experience and your book."

Ann, being my health-care agent, was definitely nervous. She said, "I was honored to be your health-care agent yet concerned your family might question any major decision if one had to be made."

MY SISTER PATTY'S THOUGHTS

I will never forget the phone call.

My Mother was on the other end of the line hysterical, telling me that my older brother Joe, whom I loved and respected, had a brain tumor. How could this be when I had just seen him a few days before at my Mom's, looking fine? The only thing he mentioned to me, in passing, was that since he had recovered from the flu, he felt some numbness in his left arm. I said, "Well, make an appointment to see your doctor; it's probably nothing, maybe a pinched nerve."

I left to go back to Cape Cod where I had been living for about six months. To help you understand what a close family we are, I had never lived further than one street away from Joe or my Mom; I became a rebel at 44 years old and moved two hours away. Two days after visiting my Mother, the phone call came, and that same day I made my way back to Waltham; the surgery would be in two days. It had been such a whirlwind that there was no time to process what was actually going to happen. My brothers and I have always tried to be there for each other. We grew up with a lot of adversity in our childhood, because of a very sick Father, but nothing could prepare us for this.

I tried to be strong for Joe until he handed me a book about sisters and said, *"If I don't make it, I want you to have this."*

I still cherish it to this day. The next day we were off to Brigham and Women's Hospital in Boston for his surgery. When the time came, I accompanied Joe to pre-op. Brigham and Women's is a teaching hospital, so they had an apprentice practicing on him to insert his I.V.'s. After three attempts I became so irate and said to the nurse, "Please do it, I can't watch this any longer." Assuming there would be a lot of suffering post-surgery, I could not bear to see him suffering now. What was so amazing is that Joe was in such a state of peace, lying there not saying a word just clutching a pair of rosary beads that our grandmother had left him. He is a man of great faith and knew that he was now in God's hands.

My immediate family, and a very dear friend Ann, settled in for what would become the longest night of our lives. There was a lot of pacing, a lot of crying and even a little bit of nervous laughter during the next twelve hours. When the surgery was over, we would wait a little longer while he was in recovery. When they said we could go in to see him we were shocked to see him sitting up, wide awake, and talking; this seemed unusual after such a long surgery.

What we would come to know, a few days later, is that Joe was suffering from an undiagnosed steroid psychosis. Joe took off all his clothes, which is contrary behavior for him. Immediately after he attempted to jump out of a window on the tenth floor of Brigham and Women's, which by the grace of God was locked and could not be opened. He then called our brother Skip and asked him to come to the hospital and kill him. When Joe's surgeon Dr. Black was notified of his behavior, he diagnosed him and weaned him very slowly off the steroids; it actually took about three weeks. It was so hard to see what he was going through but such a relief to finally know what was wrong.

While Joe was still at Brigham and Women's, Ann and I had a phone conversation with Dr. Black about Joe's prognosis. He explained to us that the surgery was much more extensive than he had anticipated because the tumor was much larger than the x-rays and MRI showed. He went into surgery believing the tumor was resting near the skull but instead found it buried in the brain with branch-like tissue infiltrating. It was also Atypical, which meant he would need grueling radiation treatment. He originally told Joe he would have some mild paralysis on his left side but was now telling us he would probably be in a wheelchair and need some rehab for about two years. It was a terrible blow to all of us, but not once did I think he would never walk again. Joe would not hear of it and, with a lot of hard work and determination, the love and support of family and friends and God's blessings, he would prove everyone wrong.

After a week in the hospital Joe was transferred to Wingate at Brighton Rehab where he would spend the next month. When we arrived I started setting up his room. Joe was a teacher, and we have a large family, so, between co-workers, students, family and friends, there were literally hundreds of cards. My O.C.D. kicked in, so I decided to display them around the room and then left Joe comfortably resting in bed. When I arrived the next morning, the room had been trashed! Every card I so meticulously displayed was pulled down and thrown around, the bed was unmade, and Joe was sitting in a pile of shredded pieces of paper. I asked him what had happened, and he said he didn't know. His psychotic symptoms were rearing their ugly head again; he felt like he was jumping out of his skin.

The following weeks were a roller coaster ride of good and bad days, but through it all Joe stayed focused, worked so hard, and defied the odds. When discussing the writing of this book he revealed to me that every specialist he worked with at rehab encouraged him to learn to manage his life while sitting in a wheelchair; he would not hear of it. He was told that no one with the extent of a tumor he had was able to walk again unassisted.

His response was, "I will defy the odds and walk out of here. I will leave on my own two feet." And he did.

Joe is considered a *medical miracle* and has lived his life post-surgery with continued deep faith, grace, and gratitude. He rarely complains about his residual issues with his left foot and is an inspiration to everyone who meets him."

CHAPTER 13
DR. BLACK—THE PERSON AND THE SURGEON

Now having read the book, I am sure that you fully comprehend my admiration for Dr. Black as a person, as well as my confidence in him as a surgeon. In his office, a map designed by the nurses represented the numerous parts of the world from which people had traveled in order to be afforded the opportunity, and the privilege, to have Dr. Black perform their surgeries. The staff utilized stickpins to designate the nations of origin of the patients, and the number of countries involved was truly amazing.

After my surgery, for the next three years, I underwent an MRI every six months to monitor the possibility of further tumor growth. Approximately a week after each scan, I would meet with Dr. Black to discuss the results. During my office visits, I often had conversations with other patients. We all came to the same conclusion that Dr. Black regards *each* patient as if he or she were his *only* patient. I recall the first words he said to Ann and me:

"If you need ten minutes, I will give you ten minutes; if you need three hours, I will give you three hours."

Delivered in his sincere, soft-spoken, and reassuring manner, these words will be forever emblazoned in my memory; it's as if one is listening to someone of the same stature as the Pope. Amazingly, prior to my surgery, Dr. Black performed an eight-hour operation, rested for an hour, and then operated on me for twelve hours.

The following is a postoperative conversation that I held with Dr. Black that I thought you might enjoy. On my head were four small bumps in a rectangular pattern. I never mentioned them until my first six-month visit.

I asked Dr. Black, "What are these bumps on my head?"

He said, "Screws."

"Screws? What screws?"

"The screws holding in the plate. How do you think your head is being kept together?"

"I never thought about it. How come you never mentioned it?"

"I tried to, but when I was explaining the surgery, marking your head and then taking out the saw, you said you had heard enough."

"I do remember stopping you midsentence; that's fair enough."

Speaking to other patients while waiting to be seen by Dr. Black was always interesting. I do not remember the order or the dates of any of these conversations, but they all took place in the waiting room.

While talking to one patient, I asked where he was from, assuming he would say he was from a neighboring city or town.

He said, "I just recently moved here from California."

"What brought you to Boston?" I asked.

He replied, "Dr. Black." He told me his physician in California said Dr. Black was the best neurosurgeon in the world, and if he could arrange an appointment with him, why would he go to anyone else?

I replied, "You made the right decision."

Another patient heard me tell Nancy Olsen Bailey to please give my paperwork to Dr. Black.

I sat down next to her, and she said in amazement, "*You have Dr. Black?*"

I told her, "I do."

She said, "You are so fortunate. I have been trying to get an appointment with him for a long time, but he's currently not accepting new patients."

I replied, "I realize how fortunate I am."

There were multiple physicians using the waiting room, and she was being treated by someone other than Dr. Black.

I spoke to another patient who was also being seen by another surgeon. When I mentioned Dr. Black was my doctor, she told me a friend of hers had a brain tumor and had been examined by five different surgeons. Each one told her the same thing: the tumor was inoperable, and she had approximately six months to live. Fortunately, she was persistent and made an appointment with Dr. Black, who told her he could perform the surgery. Three years later, she is doing very well.

There were times when Dr. Black would have an emergency surgery or was spending extra time with a patient. While waiting for my appointment, I noticed two patients becoming impatient and agitated. They were complaining about the long wait, so I assumed it was their first time seeing Dr. Black. I moved to sit beside them and asked if it was their initial visit, and it was. I told them he was my surgeon, and at times, he would have to tend to an emergency or was spending extra time with a patient. I explained to them that Dr. Black treated each patient as if he or she was his only one. He gave them all the time and attention they needed and would do the same for them, as I had personally experienced. They appeared more relaxed and relieved, realizing what I said could indeed come to fruition for them. Meanwhile, I was more than happy to be seen at 1:00 p.m. for my 9:30 a.m. appointment.

At one appointment, my brother Skip came with me. We were taken into a conference room that was outfitted with a large desk and about a dozen chairs. I was a little nervous, never having been in the conference room, but the nurse said all the other rooms were occupied. She said Dr. Black was unavailable, so we would be seen by a few of his assistants. My brother asked if he could use the phone, and she said that would be fine. He owned a construction company and had to make some phone calls.

Approximately twenty minutes later, three doctors, whom I had never met before, entered the room while Skip was on the phone. He finished his call and sat down next to me. For whatever reason (possibly because he was on the phone), the doctors assumed he was the patient and directed all the questions to him. My brother is a character and just played along.

They asked, "So how are you feeling?"

My brother said, "Very well, thanks."

"The scar has healed very well. Do you get headaches?"

"No."

"Are you having any problems we should know about?"

"No, everything is fine."

"The MRI looked clean, and you will have to have another MRI in a year."

He said, "I'm not sure why I would have to have an MRI; my brother is the one who had the surgery."

We could tell they were embarrassed, but we all had a good laugh. It was difficult to contain my laughter during this brief conversation.

To further add credence to my deep respect for Dr. Peter Black, in 2008, the Brain Science Foundation announced that he had been chosen as President-Elect of the World Federation of Neurosurgical Societies. A brochure by the Foundation reads,

> Brain Science Foundation Trustee and medical advisor, Peter Black, MD, PhD, has been elected President-Elect of the World Federation of Neurosurgical Societies (WFNS), a professional and scientific nongovernmental organization composed of five continental associations, 89 national neurosurgical societies and six affiliate societies representing approximately 25,000 neurosurgeons worldwide. Dr.

Black will serve two years as President-Elect, four years as President, followed by two years as Past-President.

Dr. Black is the Franc D. Ingraham Professor of Neurosurgery at Harvard Medical School and Founding Chair of the Department of Neurosurgery at Brigham and Women's Hospital, a post he held for over twenty years. He is consistently listed in Best Doctors in America with special interest in brain tumor surgery; image-guided minimally invasive neurosurgery; skull-base surgery; and brain mapping. With Dr. Ferenc Jolesz, he helped to develop the world's first intraoperative MRI at BWH and has used this device to improve brain tumor treatment. With the help of BSF Founders Steven and Kathy Haley, he created the Meningioma Center of Excellence at BWH.

As President-Elect of the WFNS, Dr. Black will help to lead the Federation's efforts to advance neurological surgery and all of its aspects. The organization pursues these goals by educating and training neurosurgeons around the globe and providing instruments and equipment for them. Additionally, it facilitates relationships among neurosurgical surgeons and increases the exchange of knowledge, ideas, and discussions on neurosurgical issues through education courses and a World Congress of Neurosurgery held every four years.[9]

Now can you fully understand why I had so much faith in Dr. Black?

---

[9] Brain Science Foundation pamphlet, winter 2008, page 3. Brigham and Women's Hospital Leadership Achievements by Author - Jaime Mason. www. brainscience foundation.org.

CHRONOLOGICAL LISTING OF MY TREATMENT AND RECOVERY

The following details the chronology of my treatment and recovery:

Date 1999	Nurses Needed for Assistance	Walking Aids	Hand and Arm Movement— Raised	Leg Movement— Step	Chores Performed
March 25 &26	Two	Wheelchair	Left—0 Right— 25% Movement	Left—0 Right— 25% Movement	None
March 27	Two	Wheelchair	Left—0 Right— 25% Movement	Left—0 Right— 50% Movement	None
March 28	Two	Wheelchair	Left— 1/2 inch Right - five inches	Left—0 Right— three inches[10]	None
March 29	Two	Wheelchair. Brace from foot to buttocks	Left—one inch Right— one foot	Left—0 Right— four inches	None

---

[10] In my initial steps, I measured the point at which my toe was to where my forward toe landed.

Date 1999	Nurses Needed for Assistance	Walking Aids	Hand and Arm Movement— Raised	Leg Movement— Step	Chores Performed
March 30	Two	Wheelchair. Same brace	Left—one inch Right— one foot	Left—0 Right— four inches	Ate dinner without assistance
March 31	One	Wheelchair. Same brace	Left—two inches Right— one foot	Left—0 Right— four inches	
April 1	One	Wheelchair Same brace	Left—two inches Right— one foot	Left—0 Right— four inches	Took my first shower
April 2	One	Walker with assistance Same brace	Left—four inches Right—one and a half feet	Left—two inches Right— six inches[11]	Pour orange juice Dress and undress Brush teeth
April 3	One	Walker with assistance Same brace	Left—five inches Right—one and a half feet	Left—three inches Right— six inches	Shaved
April 4	One	Walker with assistance Same brace	Left—five inches Right—one and a half feet	Left—three inches Right— six inches	Showered without nurse in bathroom
April 5	One	Walker with assistance Brace from foot to knee	Left—seven inches Right—one and a half feet	Left—four inches Right-seven inches	

---

[11] See previous note - #10.

Date 1999	Nurses Needed for Assistance	Walking Aids	Hand and Arm Movement— Raised	Leg Movement— Step	Chores Performed
April 6	No assistance from here on	Walker— on my own Same brace	Left—eight inches Right—one and a half feet	Left—four inches Right—ten inches	Get in and out of bed on my own
April 7		Walker— on my own Same brace	Left—twelve inches Right—full mobility	Left—six inches Right—ten inches	Go up and down stairs and the curb with walker
April 8		Four-legged cane with assistance Same brace	Left—twelve inches Right—full mobility	Left—six inches Right—half a stride[12]	
April 9		Four-legged cane with assistance Same brace	Left—twelve inches Right—full mobility	Left—six inches Right—half a stride	Shower with Four-legged cane I wrote in journal
April 10		Four-legged cane with assistance Same brace	Left—twelve inches Right—full mobility	Left—six inches Right—half a stride	

---

[12] A stride for a male of my height is approximately twenty-eight inches, measuring from the hind heel to the toe of the plant foot. Although I took a full stride with both legs, the stride with my left leg was shorter than the stride with my right leg because the tumor was still attached to the nerve restricting my stride with my left leg. My right-leg stride was approximately twenty-eight inches, and the left leg was approximately twenty-four inches.

Date 1999	Nurses Needed for Assistance	Walking Aids	Hand and Arm Movement— Raised	Leg Movement— Step	Chores Performed
April 11		Four-legged cane with assistance Same brace	Left—twelve inches Right—full mobility	Left—six inches Right—3/4 stride	
April 12		Four-legged cane with assistance Same brace	Left—twelve inches Right—full mobility	Left—six inches Right—3/4 stride	Get up from ground using only cane
April 13		Four-legged cane with assistance Same brace	Left—twelve inches Right—full mobility	Left—six inches Right—3/4 stride	
April 14		Same cane New brace covering foot and ankle	Left—full mobility Right—full mobility	Left—six inches Right—7/8 stride	Stood on my own lifting my cane
April 15		Same cane Same brace	Full mobility with both arms from here on	Left—six inches Right—7/8 stride	
April 16		Regular cane Same brace		Left—six inches Right—7/8 stride	Walked without assistance
April 17		Regular cane Same brace		Left—eight inches Right—7/8 stride	Walk up and down curb with regular cane
April 18		Regular cane Same brace		Left—half stride Right—Full stride[13]	Walked holding the cane off the ground

---

[13] See previous note #12 on stride length.

Date 1999	Nurses Needed for Assistance	Walking Aids	Hand and Arm Movement— Raised	Leg Movement— Step	Chores Performed
April 19		Same brace		Left—3/4 stride Right—Full stride[14]	Walked without any supportive device
April 20		Same brace		Both legs— Full stride[15]	Walked up and down curb
April 21		Same brace			
April 22		Same brace			
April 23		Same brace			Delivered a glass of orange juice to OT
April 24—27		Same brace			Carried groceries from car to house
April 28		No wheelchair, No walker, No cane or brace			

---

[14] See previous note #12 on stride length.
[15] See previous note #12 on stride length.

A MIRACLE

The medical staff spoke of me as being a miracle. I did indeed consistently and with purpose work very hard, but there were too many coincidences that occurred for me to believe that *God* did not intervene in the entire process. It seems almost impossible that all of the following events occurred at such opportune times:

I made an appointment to see my primary-care doctor immediately after my problem occurred.

I called Kathy Mulcahey, who miraculously, given the number of surgeons in Boston, was associated with Dr. Black, whom I originally wanted to see.

Kathy Mulcahey called Dr. Black's office that same morning of the day I called her.

Dr. Black returned from his vacation after I was informed by his office just two days prior that he would be out of the country for an extended period of time.

Dr. Black had an opening in his schedule to see me.

Prior to my appointment, Dr. Black had checked the schedule, and no operating room was available. In less than an hour, there had been a cancellation.

One day prior to my surgery, for the first time, a three-dimensional MRI was perfected that was more precise than the three previous MRIs combined.

I coincidently had a nurse who had worked on a different floor during my stay at Wingate exit a room at the exact time I was leaving. I would have otherwise never known the entire nursing staff was told by the supervising nurse to interview me.

God had been watching over me.

ACKNOWLEDGMENTS

First and foremost, I want to thank God for blessing me with the strength and determination needed to move forward past the boundaries created by my brain tumor. I would also like to thank Him for placing into my life family and friends whose unconditional love, support, and encouragement lifted me up and carried me through those difficult times.

I am extremely grateful to, and for the following special people. I would like to individually thank:

- my late Mother, Angie, and Father, Harry, for being constant presences in my life. My Mother continued to support me from the nursing home until she passed away on April 24, 2020, to the coronavirus.

- my brother Skip, who was always just a phone call away.

- my sister, Patty, who was with me before, during, and after the surgery—Her assistance in proofreading and editing this book was invaluable.

- my brother Chris, who biked fifty miles in my honor to raise money for meningioma research.

- Dr. Peter Black, whose "golden hands" enabled him to perform a delicate twelve-hour surgery under demanding circumstances—His temperament gave me full confidence that he was the only doctor that I would have wanted to perform my surgery.

- my dear friend Ann Ormond, whom I met fourteen years earlier while working on a political campaign—She was there for my each and every need. Her medical background and note-taking enabled me to focus solely on making the proper medical decisions.

- the late Father Charles Egan, pastor of our closely knit Sacred Heart parish, made up of predominantly Italian parishioners—He was a friend prior to my surgery and accepted the role as spiritual confidant during the entire process.

- my longtime friend and former English teacher Niel Porcaro, who assisted in proofreading and editing this book.

- the medical staff of Harvard Vanguard Medical Associates, Brigham and Women's Hospital, and Wingate at Brighton Rehabilitation Facility for assisting me with all my medical needs and the staff of Wingate at Brighton for encouraging me to write a book about my experience.

- members of my extended family and friends for your prayers, cards, gifts, visits, and transportation to and from radiation treatments and rehabilitation.

It is impossible to name all of you individually, but you know who you are. Your support, love, and kindness were instrumental in giving me the strength and encouragement to work myself back to life.

On a final note, let me say that you never know where life will lead you, but if you have individuals who walk before you, beside you, and behind you, anything is possible.

PICTURES OF FAMILY AND FRIENDS

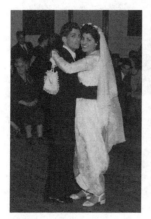

Author's parents on their
wedding day—February 1, 1948

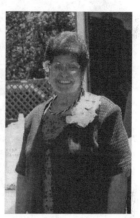

Mom with her
beautiful smile

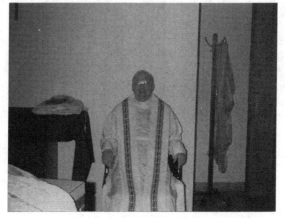

Father Egan preparing for Mass at Sacred Heart
Church in Waltham, Massachusetts

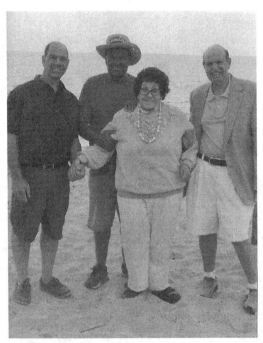

Left to right—brothers, Chris and Skip; Mom; and Author
at South Cape Beach, Mashpee, Massachusetts
Photo by Danielle LeGros

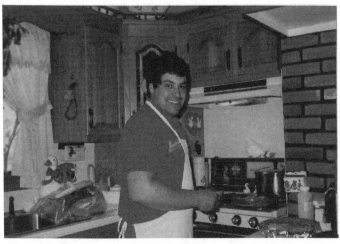

Skip cooking breakfast for Mom on Mother's Day

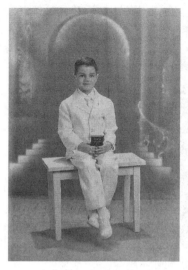 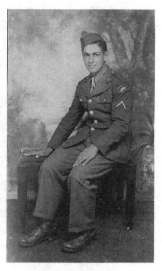

Author making his First
Communion—1959

Dad, Belmont native,
US Army World War
II veteran, and Purple
Heart recipient—1944

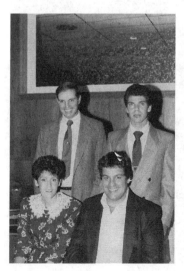 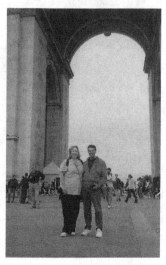

Top left to right; Author;
brother Chris; sister, Patty;
and brother Skip

Ann Ormond and Author
at Arc de Triomphe, 1998

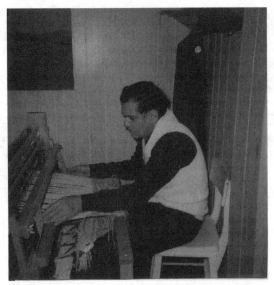

Dad working a weaving loom at the Boston Aid to the Blind

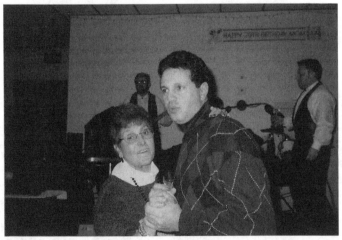

Author and Mom dancing at her surprise "seventieth birthday party"

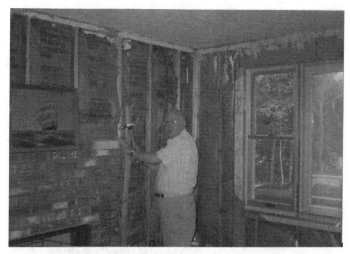

Father Egan assisting Author on building his house

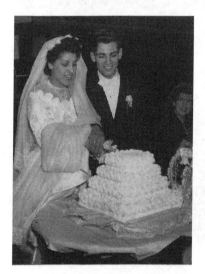

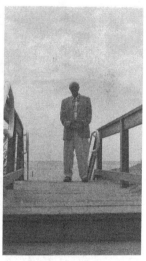

Mom and Dad cutting their
wedding cake—February 1, 1948

Author on pier at South
Cape Beach, Mashpee,
Massachusetts
Photo by Danielle LeGros

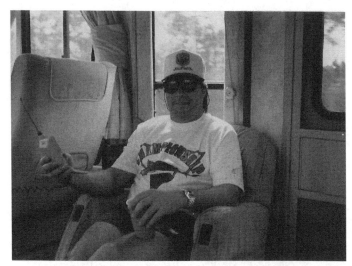

Gary Rotella en route to Tampa Bay, Florida—Super Bowl XXV

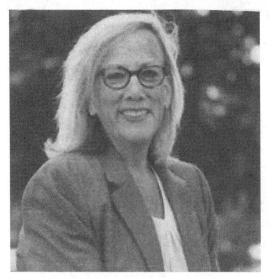

Ann Ormond enjoying life

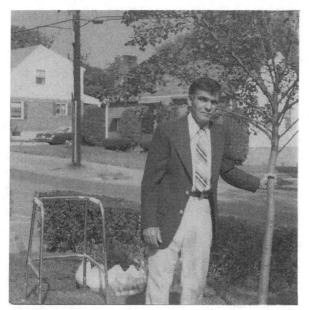

Dad walking around his front yard—Waltham, Massachusetts

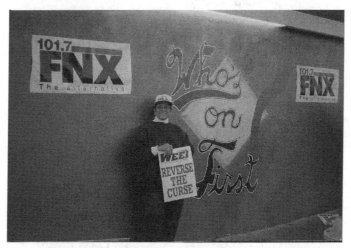

Mom and Author at Fenway Park, Red Sox game,
Roger Clemens versus Pedro Martinez

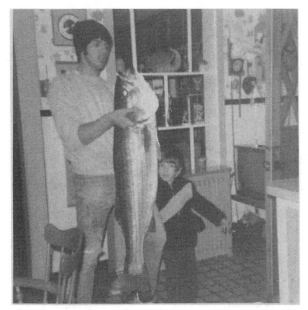

Author and brother Chris admiring a forty-pound striped bass

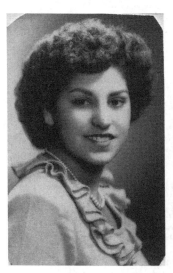

Mom in her younger days

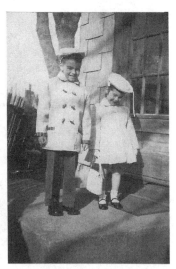

Author and his sister, Patty

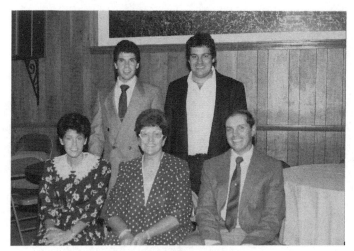

Back row left to right: brothers, Chris and Skip;
sister, Patty; Mom; and Author

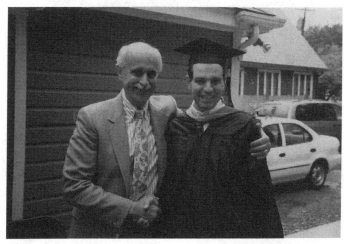

Niel Porcaro and Author at master's degree party

EPILOGUE

I returned to school in September of 1999, six months after being told I may never walk. The health teacher was amazed at my recovery. She asked if, when I had the opportunity, I would speak to her classes about my experience; I agreed to do so.

I discussed with the students the importance of living a healthy lifestyle: eating correctly, not smoking, not drinking in excess, not taking drugs, and exercising. Dr. Black was insistent that my lifestyle in my adolescent years through adulthood was an instrumental component contributing to the strength and endurance I displayed during my surgery and through my recovery.

I described to the classes my grueling workout that began shortly after the operation. It started with moving my left arm and left leg about half an inch eight hours a day. They asked what gave me the inspiration to perform that task. I said there was no other option. I knew with work I would walk again; the alternative would mean spending the rest of my life in a wheelchair. I would not hear of it. During my daily workouts, I could see progress. Each small step (literally and figuratively) was monumental because, after constantly being told you may never walk, any minor increment is like conquering a battle to eventually win the war. I strived to accomplish victory not only for myself but for members of my family and friends who supported and prayed for me during those countless hours, days, weeks, and months. My battle was not a solo flight but a team effort.

If you are in a situation like what I endured, you must believe in yourself no matter what others are telling you. It is also important to have an advocate, with whom you can be truthful and share information too overwhelming for others. It can be a friend, a family member, a counselor, or a professional. In my case, it was my brother Skip. My Mother and sister had been through enough during their life, so they didn't have to know all the particulars of each of my problems. Skip was strong enough to handle the situation.

Although there was some physical pain I endured during this ordeal, there was also the mental anguish. I have stated earlier that I am not an emotional person, but there were a number of times I cried during my recovery. Some were tears of fear and not knowing the future, and some were tears of joy for the progress I was making. I stressed to the students the importance of doing your homework and researching a doctor who could be part of your medical team. One has to have as much confidence in whomever one chooses as I did in Dr. Black. Knowledge is power in any situation in life. At the end of each class, the students stated they were amazed at my willpower and strength through the whole process.

I continued teaching until 2010, and, after thirty-three years of educating, I retired. I thoroughly enjoyed my profession and am thankful to all my friends in education who supported and assisted me through my surgery and recovery. After my retirement, I moved to Cape Cod, Massachusetts, to the home I myself built in 1987.

It does not seem possible, but twenty-one years have passed since the surgery, and I am doing very well. I have occasional minor pain and a slight limp, but nothing significant enough to keep me from living a normal life. I am enjoying golfing, fishing, boating, and clamming for my leisurely pleasure and continue to work out daily. I spend my winters in Naples, Florida, which has been a real blessing—no cold weather or heavy snow to trudge through. Through the years, I have seen a physical therapist for an ache or pain, but that's as much a part of the aging process as the operation.

As referenced earlier, I also received numerous cards, phone calls, and visitors in the hospital and nursing facility. This results from my Mother being one of twelve siblings and my Father being one of nine siblings. I had thirty-three first cousins and kept in touch with many of them. By 1999, I had taught for twenty years and coached baseball for twenty-five years. At the risk of leaving someone out, I chose not to mention all of the people who, in some fashion, gave me their love and support. Sometime after the operation, I was told that a couple of groups of my closer friends had established a phone chain and were calling each other with the results at 4:30 a.m. the morning of my surgery. I have been truly blessed to have such wonderful family and friends. With all the various forms of blessings I received, it would have been impossible to thank everyone individually. Shortly after my radiation was complete in 1999, I submitted a *thank-you* as a letter to the editor, which was printed in our daily newspaper.

I visited Wingate at Brighton in 2009, hoping to find a staff member who had worked with me in 1999. I spoke to the head nurse on the second floor, and she said that the only one still working from the second floor since 1999 was the floor custodian and that he was off that day. At the exact time I was leaving, a nurse walked out of one of the rooms. The head nurse asked her if she remembered Joe Salvo.

She said, "The schoolteacher?"

I turned around, walked back, and said, "Yes, how do you know me? I knew my nurses, and you were not one of my nurses."

She replied, "At the time, I worked on the first floor."

I said, "Then how do you know me?"

She said, "The supervising nurse at Wingate had a meeting with the entire staff and stated there was a miracle happening in room 110. We were assigned to interview you."

I said, "That explains the reason for the interviews." I never would have known the reason for all the nurses' visits and interviews if that nurse had not exited that room at the exact time I was leaving. I should have determined that something was peculiar because the nurses started their interviews the day after the head nurse asked me to walk.

Post-surgery, I was required to have an MRI every six months for the first two years. From the third to the fifth year, I was scanned yearly. Although the five-year mark without reoccurrence is not a guarantee of no future difficulties, doctors and articles in medical journals claim that it's a major milestone when you have had a brain tumor. After my fifth year, I was required to have an MRI every two years. In 2010, my MRI showed a very small dural-based meningioma tumor. As a precaution, I had an MRI every six months. In 2013, another appeared and in 2015 a third. Since there was no growth in the first two in 2015, we decided to have an MRI once a year.

My yearly scan in May of 2018 showed there was no detectable change in size of any of the three since April of 2015, so we changed the frequency of my MRIs to every two years. My most recent MRI on June 18, 2020, detected a very slight increase in size in all three tumors—approximately one-sixth of an inch. Since the scan showed minimal growth in 2020, as a precautionary measure, I plan to have my next MRI in one year instead of two. I don't dwell on this situation of the slight change. If there is ever major growth in any or all of the tumors, I will make a decision at that time on what should be done.

These three tumors are in a different area than the original tumor. Thanks to radiation applied by Dr. Jay Loeffler, the area radiated was clean with no regrowth. I mentioned earlier that only once did I have to press the bulb to signal the staff to stop the MRI. If you have not had an MRI, I can tell you it is not a pleasant experience. I believe I have had thirty-one MRIs, and other than the second MRI technician, the technicians and nurses were all very compassionate and sympathetic to the situation. At times, I felt sorry for myself, until I realized that if I were in a country where MRIs were not available, I would have never survived.

I met with Dr. Black after each MRI, and he was always pleased with my results. During one of my early office visits with him, he explained that meningiomas were fairly common. Unless you had symptoms or an MRI, they would lie dormant, and you would be unaware that you even had one. My Mother had lost sight in one of her eyes, and an MRI revealed she had two small meningioma tumors. She had also been a patient of Dr. Black's. In 2008, when he was elected president-elect of the World Federation of Neurosurgical Societies, we were assigned a new neurosurgeon.

Since the surgery, I have lost my Mom and two close friends who were all instrumental in my recovery. My friend and spiritual confidant Father Charles Egan passed away in 2003, and my close friend since childhood Gary Rotella passed away in 2015.

My Mom resided in a nursing facility about one and a half hours away from my home on Cape Cod. She turned ninety-two years old on January 25, of 2020 and as mentioned passed away on April 24, 2020. Prior to her passing, I found great pleasure in visiting her three days a week as well as engaging daily in warm and loving conversations. We had unconditional love for each other, and she is sadly missed.

I never ran the Boston Marathon, but I can still walk without the use of any assistive devices.

The following are words to live by:
Work to the best of your ability, and leave the rest up to God.

.

ABOUT THE AUTHOR

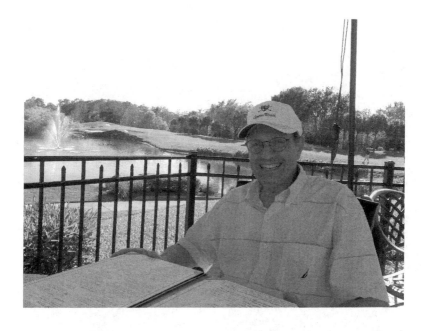

Joseph C. Salvo holds a Bachelor of Science - Management Degree from Bentley University and both a Masters' Degree in Education and a Certificate in Administration from University of Massachusetts Lowell. He is a former business teacher for seventeen years at Waltham High School and a former teacher of technology for sixteen years at Kennedy Middle School in Waltham, Massachusetts.

For the City of Waltham he was a Voter Registrar, Chairman of the Parks and Recreation Board, and a member of the Community Preservation Committee. At Waltham High School he was a varsity softball coach for twenty years and advisor to the yearbook for three years. He also volunteered for various positions in baseball leagues in Waltham. Throughout his life he coordinated and assisted with numerous fund raising activities for the sick and underprivileged. Since his surgery Joseph has coached several individuals with brain tumors through their operation. Joseph is retired and now enjoys fishing, boating, clamming and golfing on Cape Cod in Mashpee, Massachusetts. This is his first endeavor to publish a book.